Get Your Lean On

Get Your Lean On

a simple, sensible yet scientific
WEIGHT LOSS SOLUTION

TONY BEDNAROWSKI

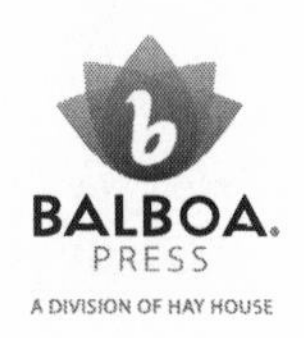

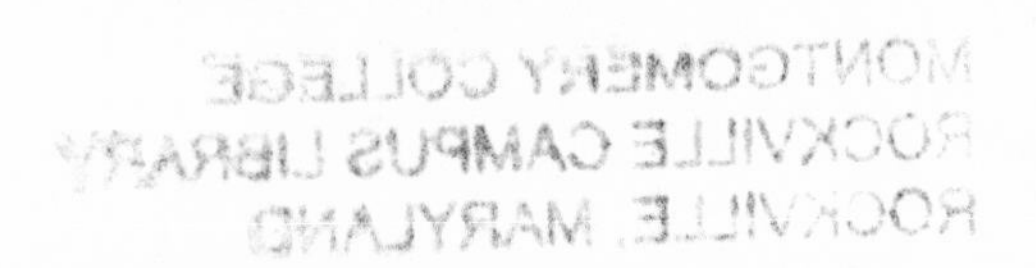

Balboa Press books may be ordered through booksellers or by contacting:

Balboa Press
A Division of Hay House
1663 Liberty Drive
Bloomington, IN 47403
www.balboapress.com
1-(877) 407-4847

Printed in the United States of America

ISBN: 978-1-4525-7003-7 (sc)
ISBN: 978-1-4525-7005-1 (hc)
ISBN: 978-1-4525-7004-4 (e)

Library of Congress Control Number: 2013904119

Balboa Press rev. date: 03/08/2013

Table of Contents

Foreword

By Jen Owen

If you take a look at the health and fitness section in any bookstore, you will be treated to hundreds of titles that all claim to be the latest and greatest approach to weight loss. Like our appetites, Americans simply can't get enough of the diet-book buffet.

We're so hungry for the end-all, be-all in weight loss success that many of us will do or try just about anything to shed a few pounds. But losing weight doesn't have to be complicated, and that's what I absolutely love about Tony's *Get Your Lean On* approach.

Tony breaks his approach down into easy-to-understand nuggets, and he explains complicated subjects in simple terms. You don't need a degree in nutritional science to understand what he's saying. He's done all the research and the work so you don't have to.

He also includes delicious recipes you can make at home. These meals do not require you to hunt specialty stores for rare ingredients, nor will they break your budget. They're easy to follow, easy to make, and frankly, delicious. It's real food for real people.

But perhaps what makes the most impact for me personally was reading all the testimonials from the many satisfied people Tony has helped over the years. Their stories are truly motivational for anyone on the same journey. They will inspire you with their candor, and their enthusiasm for their newfound healthy way of life is infectious.

Now on a personal note …

Tony is the real deal.

You will not find a more positive person. Even at some of the most challenging points in his life, he always finds the bright spot in any situation. He's also kind, considerate, funny, and thoughtful.

More importantly, Tony is also one of the most generous and genuine people out there. He's passionate about what he does, and he's passionate about helping people realize their fullest potential.

There are a million other reasons I'm a big Tony fan, but your time is better spent reading the rest of this book so you can start one of the most amazing journeys in your life.

Have fun!

—Jen

Jennifer Owen is a professional writer with more than twenty years of experience in various print and online media ventures, as well as public relations for small to mid-size business-to-business companies in the building products industry. A journalism graduate, her early career consisted of reporting and editing at weekly and daily newspapers in her home state of Wisconsin. She later transitioned to feature writing for lifestyle and healthy living publications. She currently works as a web content specialist for an e-commerce retailer.

ACKNOWLEDGMENTS

I would like to give special thanks for help in the following areas.

» Jen Owen, editing
» Shana Conradt, recipe collaboration and production
» Taylor Greenwood, photography
» Kimberly Byrne, cover design
» Brett Belau, web and social media design and marketing
» Larry Dorn, investor

Each one of these contributors is not only top notch in his or her profession but also a personal and dear friend of mine. Their expertise helped make my book go from a thought to reality.

My gratitude does not end there.

I would also I like to give a very special thanks to my children, Ryan and Courtney, and my beautiful fiancée, Gina, for always believing in me, my ideas, and my dreams. No matter how crazy my ideas may have seemed, they have always been in my corner to support and encourage me. They are truly my biggest fans.

Additional thanks to the Balboa Press and staff, a division of Hay House Publishing, and Dr. Wayne Dyer, an influential icon in my life. His many teachings have helped guide me to follow my purpose regardless of what the rest of the world might think.

INTRODUCTION

My Interest in *You*

My interest and journey into nutrition and fitness began at a very early age. I can remember as a very young boy being fascinated by muscles and reading Joe Weider's *Muscle Builder* magazine, which is now known as *Muscle & Fitness*. I would literally fantasize about having muscles like the men in that magazine. As I journeyed through life, those thoughts never left my mind. It was the beginning of a lifelong journey of fitness, nutrition, and education. It was this foundation that led me to become an accomplished bodybuilder, trainer, and nutrition expert.

Since then, over my three-plus decades in this industry, I've become the founder and developer of the *Get Your Lean On* weight-loss system, founder of BeWellCooking.com, "Inspiring personal wellness," and the co-owner/publisher of *Nature's Pathways* magazine, "Your path to healthy living." These efforts have helped me realize that my greatest passion wasn't about me and my accomplishments; it was about the stepping stones needed in life that would lead me here to deliver my knowledge and expertise to you so I can help *you* achieve your goals.

This book was written for you. I don't need the athletes or celebrities I've helped to step in and promote it because my simple, sensible, yet scientific process truly speaks for itself. I want to capture the attention of real people like you who have real struggles and are desperately looking for answers and truth. As you read through the pages of my book, you will read real written testimonials that most of you will be able to relate to. Some of you may even be able to identify yourself within their writings.

Throughout *Get Your Lean On*, I will have important information that will be relevant to my process. This book will not only map out your weight loss success but will also educate you along the way so you have a better understanding of your personal journey and the road that lies ahead. My ultimate goal is to educate, inspire, and assist you in reaching your goal and help you make this your newfound healthy lifestyle. I am very grateful and honored to have this opportunity to give you the tools and foundation to make your dream become reality. Are you ready to make your-life changing move?

A New Beginning

Chances are I don't personally know you, but it's safe to say I do know about you. You've come to me looking for answers that will make sense and a system that will work for you. There are many reasons why I wrote this book. I realized nearly two decades ago when I developed my *Get Your Lean On* weight-loss system that I had something unique to offer. My process worked wonders for hundreds of people just like you who were unsatisfied with the diets they've tried. My sole purpose was to eliminate the guesswork while encompassing education throughout the pages of my process so you have an enriched understanding of what it will take to maintain your new healthy lifestyle while breaking down the stumbling blocks. I wanted to present a well laid-out process that makes weight loss easy and achievable. Finally, this is a permanent solution to your weight-loss quest.

In the beginning, my *Get Your Lean On* system was exclusively an online program people would sign up for and follow. After a point, I realized *Get Your Lean On* was the beginning of an evolution. I knew I had so much more to offer than just weight loss, so I rolled *Get Your Lean On* into BeWellCooking.com, an online wellness community geared toward weight loss as well as chronic disease education and prevention. BeWellCooking.com is not only a place where I can blog and teach people my weight-loss method but a place for nutrition tips, facts, and recipes for diabetes, Crohn's disease, celiac, heart disease, and *more.* Some of the themes on the website are:

Bewellcooking.com

Be Well: Weight Loss

Be Well: Diabetes

Be Well: Kids

Be Well: Celiac

Be Well: Crohn's

Be Well: Heart Disease

As my journey progressed, I also became the publisher of *Nature's Pathways* magazine, "Your path to healthy living." It was after years of focusing mainly on my publication that I realized by popular request that it was time to give people my weight-loss process in a tangible product they could hold and make their own—a handheld guide or playbook, if you will, to take along on their new life journey. Thus I wrote this book—*Get Your Lean On: A Simple, Sensible, yet Scientific Weight-Loss Solution.*

GYLO Success

My journey started a long time ago when I was a child. I have always been a little overweight even though I was pretty active. I guess looking back I just never really ate very well. Through my college years, it just got worse. I ate out all the time, and the studying stress helped food become my comfort. I was also one of those girls who was a friend to all the guys—you know, great personality but not girlfriend material. I got my heart broken more than once, which also helped me find comfort in food. At my highest weight, I was 210 pounds at five foot seven.

In my mid-twenties, I started working so much that it was hard for me to eat a lot, and I lost weight just from that. I got down to 180 pounds and stayed there. Then at twenty-nine, I decided I wanted to change, and I went on Weight Watchers. I got down to 154 pounds pretty fast, but I was hungry all the time and just couldn't stand the low calories.

I started eating what I thought was more normally and gained all my weight back, plus some! I tried any and every infomercial product and diet pill, but nothing was working. I was eating so little that when I would try to eat anything normal, I would just gain more weight.

At some point, I think I killed my metabolism. There I sat with my weight once again just over 180 pounds. One day while I was chatting with a friend of mine online, she pointed me to Tony, and I started looking into it. He talked about helping re-adjust your metabolism and that his plan was not calorie restrictive. I also liked the fact that all the meals were set up for me. The meal plans looked really good and I love to cook, so it made sense to give this a try.

I could tell my metabolism started changing because I was eating more meals and more calories, but the weight started coming off. I started doing some lightweight training and cardio in addition to the meal plans. Before I knew it, four months had passed and I was down forty-four pounds to bring me to 137 pounds! I was looking and feeling really, really good about myself and what I had accomplished.

I would like to say to others who are beginning their journey that there will be some bumps in the road along the way, but please hang in there, because the end result is worth the wait. Good luck to all!

—Kristie

Chapter 1

Nutrition and Macronutrients 101

The Foundation

I wanted to start out by giving you a solid foundation to build on. Let's start at the beginning with the simple basics of nutrition so you'll better understand the *whys* behind my process.

Nutrition is based on the process of eating and converting food into structural and functional body compounds to be used for the following:

» energy
» growth
» tissue repair
» bodily functions
» performance
» maintenance
» health

What is nutrition actually made up of? Nutrition is made up of five main macronutrients. Most experts will talk about three—proteins, carbohydrates, and fats—but I add two other components to my list because they are essential to your weight loss, health, and survival. Fiber, as a component of a carbohydrate, is so vital to one's overall optimal health as well as weight loss that I include it in my list. Also, the most overlooked macronutrient of all is water, without which survival would be impossible.

Here are the five macronutrients, not arranged in any significant order:

1. Proteins
2. Carbohydrates
3. Fiber
4. Fats
5. Water

All our micronutrients or essential nutrients are derived from these five main macronutrients. Essential nutrients are nutrients that can't be produced by the body but are needed to sustain life and maintain proper body functions and optimal health. All vitamins, minerals, antioxidants, enzymes, and phytochemicals are derived from our macronutrients.

Why is good nutrition so important? It is the foundation for managing proper weight as well as preventing and even reversing many chronic diseases. It is the basis for higher energy levels, better performance, and better mental focus, as well as many psychological effects like better mood, higher self-esteem, better self-image, and a higher self-worth.

Five of the six leading causes of death in America all relate to the typical American diet or what I refer to as poor nutritional choices. The leading causes of death, in order, are the following:

1. Heart disease
2. Cancer
3. Stroke

4. Chronic obstructive pulmonary disease
5. Accidents
6. Diabetes

Diet and physical inactivity kill more Americans every year than tobacco, alcohol, and firearms put together. Yes, we have an epidemic that's growing.

Let's take a look into a typical American diet and where we're going wrong. *American diets are too high in:*

» sugar;
» processed foods;
» empty calories (foods that have little to no nutritional value);
» refined flours;
» total calories;
» saturated fat;
» cholesterol; and
» sodium.

American diets are too low in:

» protein;
» heart-healthy fats;
» fiber;
» antioxidants;
» fluids;
» potassium;
» calcium; and
» magnesium.

I am here to tell you that there *is* a solution.

Over many years I'd conducted studies with a wide variety of men and women according to height, weight, gender, and age to come up with the perfect calorie range and perfect macronutrient division to maximize metabolic stimulation for optimal weight loss while revamping blood chemistry.

The process I developed not only maximizes healthy weight loss while lowering body fat levels, but it also prevents—and in many cases reverses—many chronic diseases related to poor nutritional choices. My process has helped numerous individuals eliminate the need for medications to treat cholesterol, blood pressure, acid reflux, type-two diabetes, and other ailments tied to being overweight or obese.

Now let's take a look at each of our five macronutrients and the roles they play in our nutritional needs, weight, and optimal health.

Protein 101—Our Thermogenic Friend

Protein, the main component of muscle tissue, is needed for growth, maintenance, enzyme production, hormone production, and DNA production.

Protein is one of the five macronutrients our bodies need for proper bodily functions and optimal health and to sustain life. Protein is essential for many of the body's processes, including building and repairing tissue and making enzymes, hormones, and other body chemicals. It is an important building block of bones, muscles, cartilage, skin, and blood. In my world, we refer to protein as the building blocks of life.

Protein contains four calories per gram and is the hardest macronutrient for our bodies to disassemble and process. This makes it the most thermogenic macronutrient, meaning the most stimulating to your metabolism.

What exactly is protein made up of, and where can we find it? Protein is made of smaller compounds called amino acids, which are divided into two categories, essential and nonessential, ten of which are manufactured by the body. The amino acids manufactured by your body are called nonessential. Another ten are called essential amino acids, meaning they need to be taken into your body by an outside source, namely food.

A complete protein is a protein that contains all of the essential amino acids.

All animal proteins are complete, including red meat, poultry, seafood, eggs, and dairy products. For vegetarians, complete proteins can also be obtained through certain plants, such as soy, quinoa, buckwheat, spirulina, and amaranth.

Foods can also be combined to make complete proteins like pairing beans and rice, beans and seeds, beans and nuts, and beans and grains. When you eat hummus and pita bread, nut butter on whole-grain bread, pasta with beans, veggie burgers on whole-wheat bread, split-pea soup with whole-grain bread, or tortillas with refried beans, you are eating complete proteins. These combinations don't necessarily even have to be eaten within the same meal, so if you eat beans for lunch and rice with dinner, you've given yourself a complete protein.

Carbohydrates 101—Energy in Proportionate Amounts

The primary source of energy for all body functions, carbohydrates contain four calories per gram and are the easiest macronutrient for our bodies to process, leaving it the least thermogenic—the least metabolically stimulating. The body breaks down carbohydrates into sugar units to be used as fuel by the body's cells and muscles.

In our bodies, carbohydrates are being broken down and used as energy. When the body doesn't need to use carbohydrates for energy, it stores them in the liver and muscles, a process known as glycogen storage. It is important to know that when glycogen reserves are full, excess glycogen broken down from carbohydrate ingestion will be turned into and stored as fat. When our body needs a quick boost of energy, it converts glycogen into energy. When it needs a prolonged burst of energy, it converts fat to energy.

Carbohydrates are divided into two types: simple and complex. This is based on their chemical structure and reflects how quickly sugar is digested and absorbed.

Complex Carbohydrates

These carbohydrates are mainly referred to as starches and are made up of three or more sugar molecules linked together. These carbohydrates are found in whole grains, vegetables, legumes, fruits, and seeds. They differ from simple carbohydrates, like sugar, which are only made up of one or two linked sugar molecules. Complex carbohydrates take longer for your body to break down than simple carbohydrates, helping to maintain a steadier blood-sugar level.

Simple Carbohydrates

Simple carbohydrates are also called simple sugars and are made up of one or two sugar molecules linked together. Simple carbohydrates include sugars found naturally in foods such as fruits and milk products. Simple carbohydrates also include fruit juice, table sugar, honey, syrups, soft drinks, candy, baked goods, and all other processed and refined foods. These foods have fewer nutrients than foods with naturally occurring sugars, such as whole fruit or starches, and are absorbed into the bloodstream very quickly. A majority of these items will fall into the empty calorie category, meaning foods with little to *no* nutritional value.

Fiber 101—Huge Benefits, Zero Calories

Fiber is a component of carbohydrates. Fiber is so important that I include it as one of the five macronutrients. Fiber is the nondigestible part of the carbohydrate that can't be absorbed, therefore accounting for zero calories. Fiber is divided into two types: soluble and insoluble.

Soluble fiber comes from fruits, vegetables, oats, beans, peas, lentils, barley, nuts, and seeds. When mixed with liquid, it forms a gel, which helps control blood sugar and reduces cholesterol. *Insoluble fiber* comes from fruits, grains, and vegetables. It adds bulk and acts like a brush to clean out the colon. It helps food pass through the digestive tract more quickly and prevents constipation.

Fiber helps regulate and stabilize blood-sugar levels; lowers low-density lipoproteins (LDL), known as bad cholesterol; increases food volume without increasing caloric content, providing satiety; slows the emptying of the stomach, shielding carbohydrates and delaying absorption of glucose; speeds the passage of foods through the digestive system; stimulates intestinal fermentation production of short-chain fatty acids; and adds bulk to the stool.

You should try to consume thirty to thirty-five grams of fiber each day. Some health benefits associated with fiber are that it:

- lowers the risk of heart disease,
- helps prevent atherosclerosis,
- aids in preventing type-two diabetes,
- helps prevent diverticular disease,
- keeps you more regular,
- helps lower blood pressure, and
- aids in weight loss and weight maintenance.

Fats 101—the Good, the Bad, and the Ugly

Fat (lipids) are the most misunderstood macronutrient of all. They have really gotten a bad rap from the misinformed dieting industry. Yes, saturated fats and trans-fats should be avoided at all costs because of their health risks. But monounsaturated and polyunsaturated fats are essential to our bodies for numerous reasons and have many health-promoting aspects.

The fact is, we all need fats. Fat helps nutrient absorption and nerve transmission and serves as a storage site for our fat-soluble vitamins. They keep our blood running smooth and help carry fat deposits out of the body, helping raise HDL levels (good cholesterol) while lowering LDL levels (bad cholesterol). They are a vital part of maintaining the function and integrity of cellular membranes and are also used as a source of energy. In fact, too few of the good fats can result in chronic fatigue, obesity, and even heart problems.

Fats are not created equal. Some fats promote good health while others increase our risks of health problems. The key is to replace bad fats with good fats in our diet.

The Good Fats

Monounsaturated Fat

Monounsaturated fatty acids (MUFA) are fatty acids that have only one double bond in the fatty acid chain, with the remainder being single bonds. Monounsaturated fat is found in natural foods such as red meat, whole milk products, nuts, and high-fat fruits, such as olives and avocados. Monounsaturated fat helps lower total cholesterol and LDL cholesterol while increasing HDL cholesterol. Monounsaturated fat has also been proven to aid in weight loss, particularly body fat. Other great sources of monounsaturated fat are:

- canola oil;
- peanut oil;
- olive oil;
- seeds such as safflower, sunflower, and pumpkin; and
- almond butter, peanut butter, and cashew butter.

Polyunsaturated Fats

Polyunsaturated fatty acids (PUFA) are fatty acids made up of all double bonds in the fatty acid chain. Included in the class of polyunsaturated fat are omega-3, omega-6, and omega-9 fatty acid acids.

Polyunsaturated fat is found in seafood like salmon, herring, halibut, tuna, and other oily fish. Soy, flax seed, wheat germ, safflower, and sunflower oils are also high in polyunsaturated fats. Polyunsaturated fat, like monounsaturated fat, helps lower total cholesterol and LDL cholesterol while increasing HDL cholesterol, aiding in weight loss. Other great sources of polyunsaturated fat are:

» walnuts,

» sunflower seeds,

» sesame seeds,

» peanuts,

» peanut butter and nut butters,

» olive oil,

» soybeans,

» whole grain, and

» wheat.

The Bad Fats

Saturated Fats

Saturated fat consists of triglycerides containing only saturated fatty acids. This type of fat only has single bonds. To have an unsaturated, state there must be at least one double bond within the chain. Saturated fat is mainly found in animal products such as dairy, eggs, and seafood, as well as certain vegetable products, such as coconut, cottonseed oil, palm kernel oil, chocolate, and many prepared foods. Saturated fat raises triglycerides levels, total blood cholesterol, as well as LDL cholesterol (the bad cholesterol). Other sources of saturated fat include:

» coconut oil,

» coconut milk,
» cocoa butter, and
» palm oil.

These are all sources generally found in nondairy whipped toppings, coffee creamers, cookies, cakes, and other baked goods.

Trans Fat

Trans fat was invented by scientists to "hydrogenate" liquid oils to last longer in the food-production process and provide a better shelf life. As a result, trans fatty acids are formed. Trans fatty acids are found in many packaged and fried foods, such as French fries and microwave popcorn, as well as in vegetable shortening and hard-stick margarine. Trans fat raises triglycerides levels, total blood cholesterol, and LDL cholesterol and is the only fat known to lower HDL cholesterol (the good cholesterol). Avoid these fats. They are found in:

» cookies, crackers, cakes, muffins, pie crusts, pizza dough, breads;
» margarine and vegetable shortening;
» pre-mixed cake mixes, pancake mixes, and chocolate drink mixes;
» fried foods, including doughnuts, French fries, fried chicken, chicken nuggets, and hard taco shells;
» snack foods, including chips, candy, and packaged or microwave popcorn; and
» frozen dinners.

What to Do?

Read labels. Avoid using cooking oils that are high in saturated fats and/or trans-fats, such as coconut oil, palm oil, or vegetable shortening. Instead, use oils that are low in saturated fats and high in monounsaturated and polyunsaturated fats, such as canola oil, olive oil, and flax seed oil. Minimize using commercially packaged foods, which are high in trans-fats. Always read labels to look for trans-fat-free alternatives. Because saturated fats are found in animals products, use lean meats and lower-fat versions of dairy and cheeses, such as 1 and 2 percent or skim products instead of whole. Trim visible fat and skin from meat products.

Water 101—Essential to Every Living Cell

Water is essential for life. The human body consists of 70 percent water and provides hydration to every living cell. Water is the medium for all metabolic changes and necessary for nutrient transportation, blood flow, oxygen delivery, lubrication, waste elimination, and body temperature regulation.

Our bodies require a minimum amount of clean, pure, natural water every day to maintain a properly balanced level of hydration. Proper hydration increases cell communication, resulting in better health. Water transports chemical messengers, hormones, and nutrients to vital organs, which in turn produce substances that are made available to the rest of the body for proper and efficient functioning.

Today, too many of us drink coffee, fruit drinks, soft drinks, and other such products as a means of satisfying our thirst.

What many of us don't realize is that nearly all of these drinks in fact dehydrate the body. Good hydration is as important as good eating, and there is a minimum amount we need to maintain the level of water in our cells.

More benefits of a well-hydrated body include:

» increased oxygen availability to the cells;
» increased detoxification of the body;
» increased absorption and utilisation of nutrients;
» protection of the spinal cord and other sensitive tissues; and

- it helps rid waste through urination, perspiration, and bowel movements.

Water is also important for fat loss for several reasons:

- Water fills us up without adding any calories.
- Dehydration will degrade a person's ability to burn calories.
- Dehydration will reduce protein synthesis, which is needed to build or repair muscles.

I recommend drinking a minimum of two quarts of water per day. Obviously this amount can vary with size and activity level, but this is a good number to shoot for.

Note: If your urine is bright yellow, you are in a state of dehydration and need to drink more water.

Some interesting facts to note:

- The human brain is composed of 70 percent water.
- The lungs are composed of nearly 90 percent water.
- Lean muscle tissue contains about 75 percent water.
- Our bones are composed of 22 percent water.
- Body fat contains 10 percent water.
- Our blood is made up of nearly 80 percent water.
- Each day we must replace 2.5 liters of water through the consumption of water, beverages, and food.

GYLO Success

I have struggled with my weight from childhood on, and I just settled for believing that's the way life was for some. As I grew older, I searched for change and tried every diet plan imaginable. Most never worked, and the ones that did seemed to always restrict my calories so much that it was impossible to stay on them. I went up and down for years, never finding anything that would actually work for me long term.

A visit to my doctor put me in high gear searching once again for a way to lose weight. The news was that not only was I overweight, but my blood pressure and cholesterol were now at unmanageable limits and she highly recommended me to go on medication to get them back under control ASAP. I am totally against the thought of being on medication to bring my numbers in line. This prompted me to search for an alternative. That's when I went to Tony for help. He taught me about the *Get Your Lean On* lifestyle and assured me I would never again have to starve myself to lose weight. The lifestyle was very simple to follow, and I couldn't believe I was seeing results right away. I started at 240 pounds and now weigh 180 pounds.

I recently had a follow-up check up with my doctor, and she was ecstatic over my weight loss and blood test results. She asked me what I had been doing, and I told her about Tony's plan. She was so pleased with the results that she is recommending this to others in her practice.

I have finally found something that will work for me long term. It's worked so well for me that I now have my mother, sister, and daughter on it, and they are all seeing great results. Let me finish by saying I would have been the last person to ever consider joining a gym, but the changes I have seen and the way I feel about myself have helped me take that unimaginable step. I am now a member of a local gym and work out four days a week. I just want to say thank you, Tony, for helping me change my life.

—Roger

CHAPTER 2

DIET AND THE BODY—THE WOES

Why Traditional Diets Don't Work

THE DIETING INDUSTRY IS NOTORIOUS for great marketing schemes. Their cut-calorie approach or restrictive-calorie dieting has been a staple in our society for decades. You don't even have to change what you eat, just the amount. How is it possible to eat the same foods that got you where you are and truly believe it will be a permanent fix? To be successful with permanent weight loss and better health, you must create new habits, bottom line.

What's So Wrong with the Traditional Dieting Approach?

When you reduce calories below a level required to maintain lean body mass and meet metabolic demands, you do lose weight, but a good portion of that weight is muscle tissue. The scale is telling you things are going wonderfully, but the scale neglects to point out that if you lose muscle, you slow your metabolism. Muscle is calorie-active tissue; fat is simply stored fuel. Remember, the scale cannot tell the difference. Muscle is also the physical location where fat is burned, so if you lose weight and any portion of that is muscle, you've just crippled your body's fat-burning machine.

Also, when you are in a calorie-deprived state, your endocrine system attempts to protect you from starvation. Repeated bouts of this will coax the thyroid gland to make metabolic shifts so your body can survive on fewer calories. This absolutely guarantees losing weight will become a greater challenge in the future. Now on the flip side, when you go back to your so-called normal eating habits, you will more than likely gain all the weight you've lost plus an additional ten or twenty pounds. Yes, your metabolism has been affected, with no way to stimulate it. Most will end up becoming yo-yo dieters returning to the same system that failed before.

I know many of us hear big-name diet plans say they are sensible while others claim to be balanced, and nearly every one of them plays up the idea that they are a healthy lifestyle change. The point they miss is recognizing that if you want to boost your metabolism, you cannot starve metabolically active tissue. What you want to do is protect muscle while dropping body fat to stimulate increases in your metabolism, thus keeping your body more efficient at burning through food.

If all your attempts include a form of calorie deprivation, don't blame yourself. It all boils down to being misinformed. We are taught this by many dieting programs, so it's not your fault. You never really failed. It was the diet that failed you. If you recognize that with each perceived failure you return to the same technology that had failed you before, perhaps with a different twist or name but the same cut-calories approach, you will also recognize that you need not a repackaging of the same approach but a new approach—one that absolutely works.

If you find yourself like the millions of others who have been caught on this continual dieting rollercoaster, chances are your metabolism may need a boost. *Here are three simple recommendations to help kick-start your metabolic rate.*

Eat an Absolute Minimum of Twelve Hundred Calories per Day

While unhealthy and short lived, eating a low-calorie diet will help you lose weight, but too few calories will cripple your metabolism. As calorie depravation continues, your metabolic rate will slow as it tries to conserve energy. As your metabolism crashes, the weight you take off will eventually creep back on over time. Plus, by restricting your calories, you'll be more likely to crave and binge on junk foods.

Eat Every Three Hours

A regular meal schedule helps keep your body working to digest and absorb foods. Between breakfast and bed, aim to eat a meal or snack every three hours, and try to eat breakfast within ninety minutes of rising. People who regularly eat a healthy breakfast are more likely to control their weight. If you wait to eat until you're really ravenous, you're more likely to overeat later in the day. Also, breakfast helps fire up your metabolism after a full night of fasting (so break that fast).

Eat Protein with Every Meal

All foods contribute to the thermic effect, which means that all foods—carbohydrates, fats, and proteins—help to give the metabolism a gentle nudge higher when we eat them. But protein has the greatest thermic effect of all. In addition, protein can increase metabolism by helping to maintain and build muscle mass.

Smoothing out the Sugar Bumps

It is safe to say that many people don't really understand why our country has an epidemic proportion of people who are overweight or obese. Nearly two-thirds of the American population fit into one of those two categories. To compound this, a good portion of these individuals are heading for or already have type-two diabetes or other related chronic diseases or issues like high cholesterol, high triglycerides, high blood pressure, coronary artery disease, acid reflux, gout, and sleep apnea, just to name a few. There are also a number of emotional effects that accompany these issues, including low self-esteem, depression, social anxieties, and social isolation.

The good news is that these are all preventable and in most cases reversible through proper nutrition. I have personally helped many people dramatically transform their blood chemistry with my approach. After nearly two decades of research and development, I am proud of what I have to offer you in the way of education, support, and solutions for your healthy lifestyle needs.

One of the many things I am trying to educate you about is controlling high or excess sugar intake. Many people do not yet understand that by controlling or stabilizing your blood glucose levels, you will not only keep your weight under control but will also prevent and even reverse many of the related health issues associated with a high blood sugar level.

So let's take a peek inside the world of food. Simply put, there are six categories that all foods fall into. If a food does not fall into one of the five categories I list below, it then falls into the sugar circle. These are:

» animal products,
» nuts,
» butters,
» oils, and
» fats.

Outside of these five categories, everything else you consume is sugar in one form or another. Keep this in mind and you will make your weight loss a lot easier as well as become a lot healthier.

When choosing foods, stay away from anything that has *sugar* within the first five ingredients in its label. Also note that food manufacturers try to hide sugar with their own little language. The words *syrup*, *sweetener*, and anything ending in *ose* should be assumed to be sugar. A few other terms to be in tune with are:

- barley malt syrup,
- corn sweetener,
- corn syrup or corn syrup solids,
- dehydrated cane juice,
- dextrin,
- dextrose,
- fructose,
- fruit juice concentrate,
- glucose,
- high-fructose corn syrup,
- invert sugar,
- lactose,
- maltodextrin,
- malt syrup,
- maltose,
- saccharose,
- sucrose, and
- xylose.

Remember, your body doesn't know or care what the label says. It's all just sugar! Now let's get to a few simple facts about the body and sugar.

Blood Sugar

We have approximately ten pints of blood constantly traveling throughout our bodies at all times. Within these ten pints of blood, you need only about one teaspoon of sugar for all of your regular functions and activities. If you have more than a teaspoon of sugar floating through your blood vessels on a regular basis, the excess sugar will slow down your blood circulation by causing it to thicken, clogging up your blood vessels. This is essentially what happens when a person becomes diabetic.

Insulin

To keep the amount of sugar floating through your blood vessels at around a teaspoon, your body releases insulin whenever you eat foods that result in sugar entering your bloodstream. All carbohydrates fit this category. Sugar, most sweeteners, grains, cookies, pastries, cakes, pasta, and starchy vegetables like potatoes all lead to a release of sugar into your bloodstream. Insulin works by stimulating your cells to sponge up this excess sugar out of your bloodstream. Once inside your cells, sugar is used for energy, with any excess amount being converted into and stored as fat.

If you consistently eat sugary foods, drink sugary drinks, and/or eat too many processed carbohydrates, eventually your body will have released so much insulin that it will begin to lose its sensitivity to it. Ultimately this can lead to your cells not receiving a strong enough signal to sponge up excess sugar out of your blood. Excess sugar floating around your blood vessels is directly related to many health problems and chronic diseases, such as obesity, diabetes, high blood pressure, heart disease, stroke, and cancer, just to name a few.

If you have too much sugar floating around in your blood vessels, you likely also have too much insulin traveling through your system. Even if your fasting blood sugar level is in a healthy range, it is possible that you have too much insulin floating through your vessels, particularly if you have high triglycerides and/or are overweight. Normal blood sugar and high blood insulin can be the result of your cells losing sensitivity to insulin, which necessitates that your body releases extra insulin into your blood circulation in an attempt to stimulate your desensitized cells into sponging up excess sugar out of your blood circulation.

What's the problem with having too much insulin in your circulation? Excess insulin is known to cause:

- weight gain, since insulin promotes the storage of fat;
- lower cellular levels of magnesium, a mineral that is essential for keeping your blood vessels relaxed and your blood circulation efficient;
- an increase in sodium retention, which leads to holding excess water in your system, which causes high blood pressure;
- increased amounts of inflammatory compounds in your blood, which can cause direct physical damage to your blood vessel walls and encourage the development of blood clots, which can lead to heart attacks and respiratory failure;
- a reduction in HDL cholesterol (good cholesterol), an increase in undesirable small molecules of LDL cholesterol (bad cholesterol), and an increase in triglycerides, all of which increase your risk for heart disease; and
- a higher risk for cancer due to insulin's ability to contribute to cell proliferation.

What food and lifestyle choices support healthy blood sugar and insulin levels? Make nonstarchy vegetables the foundation of your diet. Dark green, leafy lettuce, tomatoes, celery, cucumber, cabbage, kale, Swiss chard, bok choy, zucchini, broccoli, cauliflower, and all unmentioned green vegetables are excellent choices.

Reduce or eliminate your intake of sugar and all foods that contain sugar. Some of the most concentrated sources of sugar are soda, cookies, chocolate bars, doughnuts, pastries, ice cream, and ketchup. Reduce or eliminate your use of sweeteners like molasses, corn syrup, high fructose corn syrup, pasteurized/heated honey, and maple syrup.

Don't drink fruit juices. Even freshly squeezed fruit juice taken over the long term can lead to high blood sugar and insulin levels. If you want to taste fruit, eat whole fruit, not the juice. The fiber, vitamins, and minerals that come with whole fruit help to slow down the pace at which the natural sugars from fruit enter your bloodstream.

Do activities and exercises that build or maintain your muscles. Muscle tissue acts as a storage site for extra sugar. The more muscle tissue you have, the better you can regulate your blood sugar and insulin levels.

Please pay attention and read your labels when buying foods. It could be the very thing that keeps your weight and health from cascading out of control.

The Processed Food Plague

Processed foods are foods that have been modified or altered to preserve shelf life while making them more convenient. These foods consist of many of the items that fill our cabinets, pantries, and refrigerators. Canned foods, snack foods, boxed meals, frozen meals, breakfast cereals, processed meats, sodas, and fruit juices are just a few examples of where you will find these chemicals, additives, and preservatives.

The trouble isn't just what's been added; it's also what's been taken away. Processed foods are stripped of their valuable nutrients while being modified for shelf life, taste, and texture. Things like fiber, antioxidants, vitamins, minerals, and good fats are being replaced with sweeteners, salts, artificial flavors, factory-created fats, colorings, chemicals, and preservatives.

Unfortunately, the once-good intentions that characterized the processed food industry have now developed into cheaper, more profitable ways to process food, leaving the buyer with a basket of empty-calorie foods, meaning foods with little to no nutritional value.

Today, thousands of additives and chemicals are being used by food companies to process our food. Many of them can have a devastating effect on our health as well as our weight. Below are some top processing ingredients to be on the lookout for.

Trans Fats

Trans fats are found in foods like French fries, doughnuts, baked goods including pastries, pie crusts, biscuits, pizza dough, cookies, and crackers, and stick margarines and shortenings.

Once proclaimed to be a heart-friendly replacement for butter and lard, trans fats are now being looked at as the biggest food-processing disaster in US history. Research has now revealed that trans fats are twice as dangerous for the heart as saturated fat.

Trans fats are worse than saturated fats because they not only raise the levels of LDL cholesterol (the bad cholesterol) but they also decrease HDL cholesterol (the good cholesterol). Saturated fats, on the other hand, are only known to raise the level of LDL cholesterol. Also unlike saturated fats, trans fats raise your levels of artery-clogging lipoprotein and triglycerides.

When picking products, check the ingredient list for words like partially hydrogenated, fractionated, or hydrogenated. The higher up these ingredients are on the list, the more trans fat the product contains.

Refined Grains

Refined grains, such as white bread, rolls, sugary low-fiber cereal, white rice, or white pasta will profoundly impact your weight when eaten in place of whole grains. The risk of heart disease, diabetes, and other chronic issues is highly increased as well.

Don't be fooled by deceptive claims of foods labeled with the words *multi-grain, stone-ground, 100 percent wheat, cracked wheat, seven-grain,* or *bran*. These are usually not whole-grain products. Color is not an indication of a whole grain either. Breads and other products can be brown because of molasses or other added ingredients. Often they are just the same old refined stuff that raises risk for high cholesterol, high blood pressure, heart attacks, insulin resistance, diabetes, and excess body fat.

While picking products, look for one of the following whole-grain ingredients to be listed first on the label. Also note that the fiber content should be at least three grams per serving. Remember, less on the ingredient list is always a good indication of a healthy product. The following are whole-grain ingredients to look for:

» brown rice
» buckwheat
» bulgur
» millet
» oatmeal
» quinoa
» rolled oats
» whole-grain barley
» whole oats
» whole rye
» whole wheat
» wild rice

Salt (Sodium)

Three-quarters of the sodium we consume in our diets isn't from the saltshaker. It's hidden in processed foods, such as canned vegetables and soups, frozen dinners, condiments like soy sauce steak, sauce, and barbeque sauce, fast foods, and cured or preserved meats like bacon, ham, and deli meats.

Sodium is necessary. It helps regulate blood pressure, maintains the body's fluid balance, transmits nerve impulses, makes muscles contract, and keeps our senses of taste, smell, and touch working properly. You need a little every day to replace what's lost through sweat and other excretions.

But what happens when we eat more salt than our bodies need? Your body retains fluid simply to dilute the excess sodium in your bloodstream.

This raises blood volume, forcing your heart to work harder while at the same time making your veins and arteries constrict. The combination raises blood pressure.

What to do? Try limiting your sodium intake to 1,500 milligrams per day. That's about the amount in three-fourths of a teaspoon of salt.

High-Fructose Corn Syrup (HFCS)

Compared to traditional sweeteners, high-fructose corn syrup costs less to make, is sweeter to the taste, and mixes more easily with other ingredients. Today we consume more than sixty-five pounds of it per person per year in drinks and sweets, as well as in other products. High-fructose corn syrup is in many frozen foods. It gives bread an inviting, brown color and soft texture, so it's also in whole-wheat bread, hamburger buns, and English muffins. It is in sauces and salad dressings, soft drinks, breakfast cereals and bars, processed snacks, and yes, even in some of our canned and packaged fruits and vegetables.

High-fructose corn syrup's chemical structure encourages overeating. It also seems to force the liver to pump more heart-threatening triglycerides into the bloodstream. In addition, fructose may adversely affect our body's chromium reserves, a mineral important for healthy levels of cholesterol, insulin, and blood sugar.

To spot fructose on a food label, look for the words *corn sweetener*, *corn syrup*, or *corn syrup solids*, as well as *high-fructose corn syrup*. Below are a few other processes to be aware of.

Sweeteners

Most processed foods contain sweeteners, many of which are artificial sugar substitutes containing no natural sugars, such as saccharine and aspartame.

Preservatives

Preservatives are a type of additive used to help stop food from spoiling. Sodium nitrate, nitrates, and nitrites are used to preserve meats such as ham bacon, deli meats, and hot dogs. Benzoic acid or sodium benzoate is added to margarine, fruit juices, and carbonated beverages. Sulfur dioxide is a toxin used in dried fruits and molasses. This also prevents brown spots on peeled fresh foods, such as potatoes and apples. Sulfur dioxide bleaches out rot, hiding inferior fruits and vegetables.

Refining

Refined flour has had the brown husk of the grain stripped away, leaving the white, refined starch found in white bread, white rice, pasta, cookies, and numerous other junk foods. Without the fibrous husk, refined starches are broken down quickly into sugar and absorbed immediately into the bloodstream, causing glucose levels to rise and increasing the risk of obesity and diabetes.

Bleaching

Part of the process wheat undergoes to become the white flour in popular baked goods involves bleaching. Various chemical bleaching agents are used, including oxide of nitrogen, chlorine, chloride, and benzoyl peroxide mixed with a variety of chemical salts.

Flavorings

The most common food additive and artificial flavorings comprise of a large number of chemicals. MSG (monosodium glutamate) is a very popular flavor enhancer. This enhancer has been banned from being used in baby foods but is still used in numerous other foods. As a general rule, if you don't recognize or can't pronounce the words on a label, don't buy it or eat it. Avoid products containing:

» benzoic acid (sodium benzoate);

» coloring;

» coal tar;

- MSG (monosodium glutamate);
- nitrates and nitrites (sodium nitrite);
- propylene glycol;
- refined or bleached flour;
- sulfites (metabisulfites); or
- sulfur dioxide.

Here are a few good rules to follow:

- Don't eat partially hydrogenated or hydrogenated trans fats.
- Don't eat products containing sugar substitutes, such as saccharine and aspartame.
- Avoid products with a long shelf life; the better they do on the shelf, the worse they are for your body.
- Avoid products that have been enriched. They have been completely destroyed during processing.
- Avoid food that has been genetically modified or engineered. Nearly all processed food contains GMO (genetically modified organisms).
- Avoid products made with ingredients described as natural flavoring or natural coloring.
- Avoid products with added sugar, and watch for words ending in "ose."

Fasting Facts and *You!*

When you fast, you are taking on a deliberate absence of food. Fasting is being looked at by many as a healthy process of cleansing one's system. This process is proclaimed to rid the body of so-called toxins, boost metabolism, and jump start weight loss. However, none of this is proven or backed up scientifically.

While short-term fasting (using the right method) is probably safe, long-term fasting deprives the body of many important nutrients. Extended fasting coaxes your endocrine system to slow, which in turn slows down your metabolism.

While in a nonfasting state, or normal metabolic conditions, one's body gets its energy primarily from glucose and fat supplied by the foods you ingest. Both your brain and nervous system use these macronutrients for energy as well as proper functioning. Additionally, one's body also stores energy in both the muscles and liver in the form of glycogen.

Within just hours of starting a fast, dietary glucose (your main energy source) is used up. When this happens, your body draws on its stored reserves. Once these reserves are exhausted, your body passes into an altered metabolic state. While in this state, your body turns to its own protein to make glucose for brain and nervous system functions. Without the proper supply lean proteins and healthy fats, this will result in a considerable breakdown in lean muscle tissue and the production of ketones. This is a very unhealthy and undesirable state to be in.

Although you will most likely lose weight, it will be due to water loss, dehydration, and muscle tissue wasting. This state will most likely be accompanied by feelings of fatigue, as well as dizziness.

After years of abusing the body with poor nutritional habits, a fasting state is not the answer for weight loss or better health. Your body is truly craving proper nutrition, including whole grains, fresh fruits and vegetables, low-fat dairy products, healthy fats, lean meats, fish, beans, and other protein sources. Then and only then can the body's systems work together effectively and efficiently. A healthy diet derived from these food choices will result in improved energy and overall health.

GYLO Success

I started Tony's plan in March, and by that September, I had lost forty-three pounds. When I started, I made a commitment to myself to stick this out and see what it would do. Staying committed and following

Tony's plan all the way through paid off! I have more energy, and for the first time in my life, I feel like I can do anything! I was always overweight, but now I weigh less than I did thirty-two years ago.

Altering your eating habits may not seem easy at first, but gradually because of the delicious food, the amounts, and the ease of system, it really makes the lifestyle something I could live with. Thanks, Tony!

—Mike

Did You Know?

In the "Did You Know" section, you will find a variety of interesting tips and facts that will enlighten you by bringing truth to the subject.

Burn Baby Burn!

Did you know that a pound of muscle burns thirty times more calories than a pound of fat. That's why it is absolutely essential that we preserve our muscle mass while ridding our body of those undesirable fat pounds.

Visualize Your Success!

Visual images can be a very powerful tool when helping achieve a goal. There are lots of creative ways to use this motivation technique, such as posting images of your goals where you will see them often. This will help you stay focused by keeping your goal fresh in your mind. Use a personal diary to measure your progress. Write down your successes as well as pitfalls to reflect upon. Also, display before and after pictures of yourself. These are all great ways to constantly remind yourself of the commitment you have made to yourself.

Ice Water—Did You Know?

Water helps reduce fat deposits and rids your body of toxins. But did you know that drinking just ten twelve-ounce glasses of water a day cooled to 40 degrees Fahrenheit will burn as much as two hundred calories? That's the equivalent of jogging three miles! It does this by taking energy to heat the water up to your body temperature. Add a lemon to the mix to help keep your blood sugars in balance.

Trying to Starve Fat Away?

Did you know that when you go on a limited-calorie diet or go for long periods of time between meals, your brain senses starvation and sends a signal to your body to store fat because famine is on the way! That's why so many people who go on these extreme fasts or extremely low-calorie diets don't drop the weight they set out to lose and actually end up storing more fat as a protective mechanism.

To drop weight (body fat), you absolutely have to keep your body from switching into starvation mode. The only way to accomplish this is by eating frequent healthy meals and snacks!

Meal Replacements

Many meal replacement shakes or bars lack sufficient fiber and phytochemicals, which aid in disease prevention as well as weight loss. In my professional opinion, these products should be used in conjunction with whole foods only and not as a replacement for food. My only recommendations on using shakes or bars is pre- and post-workout, with the remainder of your nutritional needs coming from balanced meals that provide sufficient calories, protein, fiber, and phytochemicals throughout the rest of the day.

Salt Terms and Meanings—What's Really in the Shaker?

- » **Salt or Sodium free**—less than 5mg of sodium per serving.
- » **Low Sodium**—140mgs or less of sodium per serving.
- » **Reduced or Less Sodium**—25 percent less sodium than a food's standard serving.

» **Light Sodium**—50 percent less sodium than a food's standard serving.
» **Unsalted or no Salt added**—no salt added during processing but could contain naturally occurring sodium.

Can I Spot Reducing Fat?

Unfortunately, contrary to what you've heard or want to believe, it is physically impossible to reduce fat in a specifically targeted area of your body. Body fat is reduced in layers and not in areas. So for example, doing crunches will strengthen your midsection but will not take the fat off your stomach. Similarly, an activity like walking or running will burn fat all over your body, not just in your legs or butt area. However, you can incorporate a sensible exercise program that fits your lifestyle along with your new healthy eating habits to speed up your weight loss while toning your body.

Changing Your Approach!

Changing the way you approach weight loss can help you be more successful at losing it. Most people who try to lose weight focus on one thing: weight loss. However, if you set goals, begin to eat healthy foods, become more physically active, and learn how to change behaviors, you have a true recipe for success. Over time, these changes will become routine and part of your everyday life.

Targeting Your Heart Rate

Here is a formula to find your "target heart rate" to maximize your fat burning potential:

220 - (Your Age) = (X) * .8 = target heart rate

Example: 220 - 35 = 185 * .8 = 148 beats per minute

Tip: If you also do some type of weight training, *always* do your cardio workout afterward. This is because during your weight-training session, you burn up muscle glycogen. This leaves your body searching for an alternate source of fuel when it comes time to power through your cardio workout. This alternate source of fuel will come directly from your fat storage, thus burning a higher ratio of body fat at a quicker rate.

Women and Weight Lifting—Myth or Truth?

Is it true that lifting weights causes women to bulk up? Our society seems to associate weight training with oversized muscles, which is extremely difficult for even most men to achieve.

While on a weight-lifting program, the right hormones are necessary to bulk up. Women's testosterone levels are much lower than men's, making it nearly impossible for them to build large muscles. In fact, since muscle takes up less room than fat, women tend to lose inches when they strength train. In addition to the physical benefits of increased metabolism, decreased risk of osteoporosis, and increased strength, strength training will help women slim down as well. Women, in fact, are more likely to tone up from strength training rather than bulk up. Women can actually add up to 30 percent lean muscle and end up looking thinner, feeling stronger, and being firmer.

Women with an intense fear of becoming large as a result of weight training are at a disadvantage when it comes to their health. The problem most women run into isn't building too much muscle but not building enough. This sets them up for increased risk of osteoporosis later in life, as well as a reduction in muscle mass of about 2 to 5 percent per year, which has an adverse effect on metabolism and can result in weight gain.

Are You Really Choosing Low Fat?

There are tricks to food labels that are worth knowing. Here are the food-labeling specifications developed by your very own USDA. Here is what it means when they use the terms *fat free, low fat, reduced fat, light/lite, lean,* or *extra lean*:

» Fat Free: A product contains a tiny amount of fat, 0.5 grams or less per serving.

» Low Fat: A product contains no more than 3 grams of fat per serving.

» Reduced Fat: A product contains 25 percent less fat than the original product.

» Light/Lite: A product contain 1/3 fewer calories or 1/2 the fat of the original product.

» Lean: A product contains less than 10 grams of fat, 4 grams of saturated fat, and 95 milligrams (mg) of cholesterol per serving.

» Extra Lean: A product contains only 5 grams of fat, 2 grams of saturated fat, and 95 milligrams (mg) of cholesterol per serving.

Are You Unsure about Something You Are Eating?

Could it be bad for you, your weight, or your health? When looking at labels, stay away from these five ingredients:

» simple sugar (sugar)

» enriched, bleached, or refined flour

» maltodextrin

» high-fructose corn syrup (HFCS)

» hydrogenated or partially hydrogenated oil

The Skinny on Skipping Meals to Lose Weight!

Reducing our food intake is what we've been taught to believe is the right approach to losing weight. Unfortunately, this logic undermines the intricate engine that is our metabolism. Skipping meals will actually trigger your body to slow its metabolism to save yourself from starvation. Most won't even realize it's happening until the plan backfires. Always eat three balanced meals accompanied by healthy snacks between meals each day. Make sure to include a solid protein source with each meal to properly rev up your fat-burning machine. Your best plan of attack is to shoot for eating something every three hours.

Can Diet Foods Help You Drop Pounds?

You may be surprised when I tell you that in most cases, you're doing yourself more harm than good. Scanning labels for the lowest calories and fat counts isn't necessarily the better choice. Prepackaged diet foods can have a lot of sugar and trans fat added to them.

As with carbs, it's the quality of the fat, not the amount, that makes the difference. Monounsaturated fats found in nuts, olive oil, and avocados and the polyunsaturated variety in soybean and safflower oils help your cardiovascular system, improve weight loss, and are crucial for absorbing fat-soluble vitamins and minerals.

The Scale vs. Your Progress; Get a Clearer Picture!

When using the scale as your directional indicator, remember these three important tips so you are certain you're getting an accurate reading.

1. Weigh yourself only one time per week.
2. Weight yourself on the same day every week.
3. Weight yourself first thing in the morning on an empty stomach.

Remember that weight loss comes in unpredictable spurts, so don't get frustrated if you have a week or two with no weight loss; it's just your body making normal adjustments that are necessary for progress to continue.

A person's weight can fluctuate five or more pounds throughout the day, so by following these three very simple but important rules, you will not only keep yourself from becoming frustrated by daily fluctuations but will also get an accurate picture of how your true weight loss is going.

Are Detox Plans a Good Weight-Loss Solution?

Excess weight is due to fat deposition, not a buildup of toxins. There are many detox diets. Some recommend a water fast through the day, some recommend just fruit or vegetable juices, and others allow only specific foods. Most detox diets are very low in calories; following such a diet for a few days will result in loss of the body's water and associated glycogen stores, as well as breakdown of some fat deposits. This can be highly motivating in the early stages of weight loss. However, be prepared for weight loss to reverse when you stop following a detox plan, as the body will work to restore its important glycogen stores, which are a natural and healthy part of body composition.

Fat Metabolizers—Do They Really Work?

Fat metabolizers or fat burners are a group of over-the-counter diet pills or aids with active ingredients that theoretically raise one's metabolism to help burn body fat. Despite extravagant claims, there is no scientific evidence these fat metabolizers work. Furthermore, there are serious concerns about the health risks associated with the ingredients found in a lot of these products. Known common side effects linked to some of these products are high blood pressure, severe headaches, heart rate abnormalities, seizures, heart attacks, and even deaths in some susceptible individuals.

Can Certain Foods Burn Fat?

No food can burn fat. Although there are certain foods that can help increase your metabolic rate—the rate at which your body burns calories—for short durations, it is not enough to cause noticeable weight loss. The best way to lose weight is to eat frequent nutritious meals in conjunction with some form of physical activity.

CHAPTER THREE

KEEPING IT REAL

Real People Real Stories

GYLO Success

I had wanted to lose ten to fifteen pounds for quite some time, not only to feel and look better but to be healthier. I contacted Tony about his GYLO program. I had met an acquaintance who had done the program, and he told me how much weight he had lost. He said it was really all about the food we eat, not dieting and exercise. Exercise tends to scare people off, including myself.

So I decided to give it a try. I was amazed and very pleased after the first week; I had already lost six pounds. And believe me, I was never hungry. In the two weeks that I followed it, I was down twelve pounds and my blood pressure medication was cut in half. In addition, I also bought a Gazelle and started to exercise. I have been able to add in more food groups and maintain my weight.

I would like to express a grateful thank you to Tony for

devising this new lifestyle of eating. If I can do it, anyone can. By the way, I am seventy years young and feeling great!

—Shirley

GYLO Success

I've been concerned with my weight for many years now, not just because of my appearance and the added stress on my joints but more because of my health. I have had high blood pressure since high school, and as I have gotten older, my health started to deteriorate to the point that I was taking Lipitor, Tricore, Niaspan, Allopurinol, and Availed (in all, about $600 worth of medication every three months).

My doctor had been telling me for years that I needed to lose at least fifty pounds—and preferably closer to eighty pounds—and start looking at healthy eating options to get my health back in line. I did try, but with no clear direction on how and what to eat, it was really just a lost cause.

I looked into a few different diet plans but again had no real success with them. Then I stumbled upon the Atkins diet. I started working with it and was losing weight, about thirty-five pounds in around five months, but when I went to my doctor to get my blood work done, he told me to drop that diet plan immediately. It had my triglycerides and cholesterol off the charts, putting me in a very dangerous situation.

My doctor then stepped in and asked me if I would try one of the facility's health-care dieticians. I was running out of options, so I agreed to give it a try. I went to her with an open mind, and she set me up on a diet plan. But after a short time of eating what she set up for me, I realized I was never going to be able to live on that small amount of food without feeling like I was starving to death. Once again I was back to square one and on my own.

After finally almost giving up and living with what looked like not too long a life, I found Tony. I talked to Tony personally and explained that I wanted to lose sixty to eighty pounds, but my real concern was my health and reducing or possibly getting off all the meds I had been taking for years. He gave me great confidence that, if I followed his plan, my goals were certainly within reach.

I started his process on May 28, 2007. It was easy to follow and never left me hungry—and that's very important to a guy who's six foot six and 345 pounds! In the little over four months I've been on the plan, I have lost fifty-four pounds, but the really amazing thing is that I didn't only reduce my medications … I *totally eliminated* them.

My doctor, pleased with the results, has taken me off of everything! In all his years of practice, he has never witnessed anyone's blood chemistry change that dramatically from anything other than medication. I seriously haven't felt this great in many, many years. My joints feel so much better too. I can do things I haven't been able to do without pain in quite some time.

I would just really like to say thanks to Tony for helping me drop weight and regain my health. I am currently a little over halfway to my target weight and looking forward to the day when I reach that part of my goal also.

—Steve

GYLO Success

I had tried everything under the sun from the *Stop the Insanity* diet to Weight Watchers. Some of them worked for a while, but none of them compare to the *Get Your Lean*

On system! I will admit my body was not happy with me for giving up all the sugar, starch, caffeine, and salt. It was a tough first week, but once I found out that how much weight I lost in just a couple days, it gave me the added "oomph" I needed to get through the week. I lost a total of eight pounds in the first two weeks and was really excited about the weight loss.

Since then it's been a breeze! My husband and my son are doing it with me, and we're all enjoying the benefits. My husband has lost forty pounds, and I'm down twenty-five! I'm amazed at not only the weight loss but the fact that we don't crave for anything! We're not hungry, don't have cravings, and don't feel deprived. Tony's plan is amazing! Thank you so much!

—Brenda S.

GYLO Success

I was always active and in good shape in high school. Once the college days rolled around, I found myself completely caught up in the college lifestyle, with lots of fast food, parties, and late-night snacking. The pounds slowly started creeping up on me, and before I knew it, I had put on nearly sixty pounds. I had always thought about doing something about it and had tried a few diets but could never seem to stick to one.

About a year ago, I was out shopping and ran into an old friend I hadn't seen since the high school days. We started chatting and reminiscing about the days gone by when all of a sudden, out of the blue, she congratulated me and asked when I was due. I almost fell over and died right then and there. I was so embarrassed that I didn't know what to say, so I went along with it, made up something, finished up our conversation, and went on my way. At that moment, I knew I couldn't ignore the truth any longer, and it was time to do something about the situation I had gotten myself get into.

A friend of mine directed me to Tony. His plan sounded interesting, and I liked the fact that I didn't have to take the time to measure or weigh anything and didn't have to keep track of calories. It seemed very easy to follow, and there was no guesswork involved. Everything was completely laid out for me; all I had to do was follow it. It seemed simple enough, so I made a commitment to give this plan a fair shot and set a goal to get back down to my high school weight of 140 pounds. I started the plan and still remember within the first three weeks I had already lost about twelve pounds, which really kept me motivated. Seeing the weight come off just made me want to start getting more active, so I started walking a couple days a week.

Within five and a half months, I had dropped fifty-three pounds and had reached my goal. It has now been over a year since then, and I can't describe the way I feel about myself inside. Not only do I feel great about the way I look, but my social life has completely turned around. I can honestly say I love my new lifestyle and am grateful I found my way to it. I still continue to walk and have recently started taking an aerobics class a couple times a week as well. Thank you so very much, Tony. What a difference a year can make!

—Jennifer

GYLO Success

My name is John; I have been Tony's plan for about two years. I started this lifestyle change at about 283 pounds, and my goal was to lose fifty pounds. In the first eight weeks I lost twenty pounds. Since then I have reached my goal and continue to make this my lifestyle. The menus and the meal planner are all very easy to use. The meals are very tasty, and I found out you don't have to be hungry to lose weight and be healthy.

Before this plan, I was trying to put together how to eat and be healthy by asking people questions doing certain so-called diets, and nothing seems to work like this. When I suggest it to people, I always say, "Try it for a while and see what happens. The only thing you have to lose is weight." My favorite recipes are the green turkey chili and the spaghetti squash and turkey casserole.

—John

GYLO Success

After making the commitment to follow Tony's lead, not only did I achieve the results I was looking for but I went beyond them. I am down over 130 pounds for over five years now. Thank you so much, Tony!

—Mark

GYLO Success

For the last three years, I have tried without success to improve my physical condition. Seeing myself in family pictures actually made me embarrassed of the condition I had let myself get into. No matter how hard I tried or how much my family tried to support and encourage me, I just could not stick with a diet and exercise plan. At the time, I didn't realize it, but some of the fad diets my wife, Tara, and I tried were actually hurting our bodies more than we could have imagined. I always felt tired and weak, which made it easy to put off or come up with an excuse to not exercise.

In January of 2009, I ran into Tony, whom I have known for years, although not very well. I knew Tony had competed in body-building competitions, and I had heard that he was now the owner of an Internet-based nutrition company, but I really didn't know what it was all about. While I talked with Tony, we discussed exercising and what it takes to get physically fit. Tony said to me, "Ric, it all starts with nutrition. You don't put regular unleaded into a Ferrari and expect it to perform well; you put top-grade fuel in it. If you want your body to look like a Ferrari and perform like one, start by using the right fuel."

The fuel analogy worked on me. The next day, my wife and I checked out the Tony's website and were impressed with what we saw. The meals were all set up and gave us daily meal options so we never felt like we were eating the same old, tired menu. I have always been a meat and potatoes guy and a real picky eater, so at first some of the recipes were not appealing to me. However, after trying some of the more common meals, I realized that eating healthy could taste good and fill you up, so I got a little more adventuresome and tried more of the recipes.

I never once have had to limit the amount that I eat, nor have I felt hungry shortly after eating. In fact, I have found that by eating the nutritious meals and snacks that are all laid out for you in the program, your body burns fat instead of storing it and you can actually eat yourself thinner.

My family and I have now been on the program for four months, and the results are obvious. We all feel better and look better, and now we all have the energy to exercise. It is funny to think that just four months ago I was an overweight junk food junkie, and now even though a cheat day is available, I no longer want those types of food. Potato chips and other junk food truly are like regular unleaded gas, and my body now knows it.

All I can say is thank you, Tony. You have changed my life and more than likely saved me from a heart attack.

Best of success.

—Ric

GYLO Success

I have been heavy for most of my adult life, always looking for a special diet or pill to lose weight, but I never could succeed. I really wasn't happy with the way I looked, so I just never looked.

I guess the important thing was that not only was I heavy-set, but my blood pressure was high and so was my cholesterol. That's where Tony's plan came into action for me. I had heard about Tony through a friend of mine. He told me how much weight Tony had helped him lose and how he had even eliminated his blood pressure and cholesterol medication, so I thought I would give Tony's plan a try. What did I have to lose besides maybe some of my weight? I had the potential to become the person I always wanted to be—happy and healthy.

So I went on Tony's plan, and much to my amazement, the weight just seemed to fall off. Within about six months, I was down sixty pounds and went from wearing a size eighteen pants to a size ten to twelve and am looking pretty darn good. My blood pressure and cholesterol are even back in line! I now have people complimenting me on my weight loss and asking me what I did!

All I can say is thanks so much, Tony. Believe me, it works; I'm living proof!

—Kathy

The Eighty/Twenty Rule

This is a somewhat touchy subject for me to cover, but I'm asked about it so often I feel it is imperative to include it in my book. We've all heard of the eighty/twenty rule. This rule can be applied to many things in life, including economics, business, marketing, health care, and even relationships. But what does it actually mean when applied to weight loss?

The truth is, I am an exercise enthusiast who frequents the gym five hours a week even though my competitive days are long over. As you've probably noticed, even though I am a master trainer as well as a nutrition expert, I don't really talk about exercise in my book, but there is a method behind my madness. First, please don't misunderstand; I don't want you to believe exercise does not play an important role in leading a healthy lifestyle. Exercise and physical activity are important to a healthy lifestyle and have many health-promoting aspects. Along with the health benefits, it can help speed your weight-loss process.

The reason I don't talk about it here is because I am nearly 100 percent certain that exercise or some form of daily physical activity will naturally become a part of your overall maintenance plan. You see, I've been doing this for so long that I am so confident in your willingness to find your way to become more physically active that I don't even have to stress it.

That said, the eighty/twenty rule certainly does apply here; 80 percent of your weight loss success will come directly through your nutritional choices, and 20 percent will be aided by your activity level. Yes, that is correct; the biggest impact on achieving your weight-loss goal will undoubtedly come from your nutritional choices. In fact, after more than twenty years of helping people achieve their weight-loss goals, I rarely ever had to try to convince someone to incorporate an exercise plan into the equation. Once I get people on the right track nutritionally and they start to see the weight come off, nearly 100 percent of the time they naturally migrate to some type of exercise plan and become more physically active. It's truly amazing to witness this process and watch people evolve into a whole new lifestyle all from changing what they put into their body.

Physical Activity and Exercise

Physical activity is different from exercise. Physical activity is defined as being active throughout the day by not leading a sedentary lifestyle, whereas exercise is a planned activity, such as running, cycling, aerobics, and strength training. Physical activity will become effortless once you've actually seen and felt change taking place. On the other hand, when looking at incorporating some sort of exercise program into your newfound lifestyle, please take it slow, especially if you've been inactive for some time or have never exercised before. Don't take the all-or-nothing approach. Incorporate a sound plan, and adapt it to your personality, lifestyle, schedule, and disposition. This way you will incorporate it into your lifestyle and make it a permanent placement.

Dealing with a Setback

I want to keep everything upbeat so you are getting the most out of the information I am supplying when it comes to successful weight loss and building your healthy lifestyle, but I also realize there will be setbacks. Anyone who has ever set out to achieve a goal has also had to deal with them. In fact, they are normal and in most cases necessary. They teach us things about ourselves, reinforcing and strengthening our knowledge and awareness. The problem isn't in the setback itself; it's how we choose to handle it. There are various things that can ultimately trigger a setback. These triggers will vary from person to person, so recognizing yours will help you avoid having to deal with them repeatedly.

Let's look at some common triggers while on a weight-loss plan:

» anger and frustration
» boredom
» celebrations

- » feeling overwhelmed
- » going out with friends
- » holidays and other family get-togethers
- » loneliness
- » restaurants
- » seeing a gain on the scale
- » seeing a loss on the scale
- » stress and anxiety
- » the smell or sight of baked goods
- » vacations

Each of these can set you up in a situation that may send you searching for comfort or weaken your self-control. They are each connected to an emotion that can side-track you.

Losing weight and sticking with the process calls for self-control and commitment. It is not uncommon for people to slip up from time to time. In fact, in the latter part of my process, I allow slip-ups or what I call cheats in moderation. If it happens before you get to your goal, please don't beat yourself up and think all your hard efforts have been lost.

Instead of throwing the baby out with the bathwater, consider taking these steps to overcome the setback you've been faced with.

First, own it; admit to yourself that what you have done was not in your best interest. While an occasional slip-up is not uncommon, you want to get yourself in the right frame of mind to avoid slipping back into old, familiar habits.

Second, consider the trigger that set you off. Try to figure out what made you do what you did. Perhaps it was a situation you encountered, the smell of a food, a slight weight gain, a celebration, or simply just boredom. Whatever the case, recognize and identify with it so you can avoid a future encounter.

Finally, forgive yourself. Slipping up only proves you are human. The mistake isn't the biggest part of the problem. Again, it's the steps you take afterward to recognize and avoid situations that can make a setback happen that matters most. Let the error go, and resolve to stick with the process and re-focus yourself on the goal you have set. A setback doesn't mean your goal is unattainable.

As much as most people would like it to be, weight loss is not an overnight adventure. To realize healthy, safe, and lasting changes, time is required. How long the process will last depends a lot on your starting weight, your goal, and personal persistence to sticking with the plan. Occasional detours can sometimes become part of the journey. Just make sure to clear your mind and get back on track when a setback gets you sidetracked.

Dining Out Tips 101

When watching your weight, dining out can be a challenge! Many of us dine out more than we ever have in the past, and there are more restaurants than ever available to us. With all of the different options to choose from, two things seem generally consistent: portions are large, and meals are loaded with starches and fat, which are high in sugars and calories. However, since there are so many people trying to follow more healthy lifestyles, restaurants are becoming more accommodating to your health needs than ever before. Here are some simple precautionary steps to take when going out for a meal.

» Avoid fried and battered foods. Instead, ask for special requests. Most restaurants are accommodating and will prepare your meal as you like. Ask for grilled, broiled, roasted, or steamed meats and vegetables. Requesting a side of steamed vegetables, salad, or brown or wild rice instead of French fries or other fried sides can help cut calories and fat while increasing your intake of healthy nutrients!

- When ordering salad, order your dressing on the side to limit your sugar, fat, and calorie intake. However, be careful not to pour all of the dressing provided over your salad, as it is often more than you would normally get on a salad with the dressing already on it. Depending on how hungry you are, a salad may be enough to satisfy your appetite, but make sure it includes some lean meat or fish for protein!
- When considering soup, go for the healthier, low-fat, broth-based options that are loaded with vegetables such as kidney, black, pinto, or garbanzo beans and whole grains such as barley. Avoid cream-based soups and chowders.
- Avoid all the extras, as these calories add up quickly: bread and butter, sweetened drinks, appetizers, side items, and desserts. Instead focus on a healthy balance of lean proteins, low-fat carbohydrates, and vegetables.
- Limit yourself to one alcoholic drink. Alcohol, whether in the form of a cocktail, wine, or beer, can weaken you from exercising thoughtful moderation with your food. Plus, it dehydrates you and offers no nutritional benefit. When you go out, order water instead.
- Since the body uses alcohol for energy first, followed by carbohydrates, protein, and fat, when you drink and eat, the excess calories are often stored as fat. To keep the pounds from piling on, skip higher-fat entrees and concentrate on lower-fat items, such as fish, pork, poultry, or lean cuts of red meat when having wine with dinner.
- End your meal with refreshing green or herbal tea. Ginger tea can help with digestion, and green tea is good for your overall health. Many restaurants now offer a variety of exotic teas, so treat yourself! Some teas are so fruity that they're a perfect replacement for dessert.

GYLO Success

First, I would just like to say I am so happy I took that first step! Yes, my life is truly changing! When I wake up in the morning, I feel rested and ready to go! I don't feel depressed, and I don't want to roll over and fall back to sleep! It's an amazing feeling I have never experienced before.

I have gained endurance, and my energy level is soaring. I can exercise without making excuses and feel excited about how good it makes me feel.

Looking at the big picture, I still have a ways to go, but I can feel my body changing. My clothes are fitting differently, and people are taking notice and complimenting me on the way I look. I have new energy, new motivation, and new love for life! The weight is coming off, and that is great, but the way I feel means so much more to me than any number the scale can show me.

I never thought I could feel this good. Thank you, Tony. I know this journey is going to bring me to an amazing place. I am excited to see where I will be a year from now. I feel like I am capable of accomplishing anything. It has put me in a better place mentally and physically. I feel alive!

—Kim

Chapter Four

Welcome to the Tiers of Success

About the Process

FIRST, I WANT TO MAKE sure you understand what my process is not. My process is not a diet program. Diet programs are proven not to work and for a very good reason. It's all about marketing. Most diet programs are set up to fail so you keep going back and trying it over and over again. The approach I have laid out is a simple, sensible, yet scientific process that will take you on a journey of education about food facts and smart meal planning.

It is all about what you eat! It is a process of education while eating a lot of good food! Learning the ***why*** *is the key to success.*

This journey was designed to make you aware and teach you the process of making healthier and wiser decisions when it comes to food, eating, and meal planning. Although my process is in a simple-to-follow format, I also want to make sure you are being educated along the way so when you are done with my book, you have a solid understanding of what it will take to maintain your new healthy lifestyle. You will not only lose the weight you want to lose, but it is so successful that you will make a lifelong commitment to keep it off.

You will lose the weight you desire while never being hungry.

To be successful in losing weight and keeping it off, you first must have a process you believe in, understand, are committed to, and are enthused about. Most people never reach their weight-loss goals because their method usually revolves around the all-too-forbidden cut-calorie approach. They start out with good intentions but soon realize they will never be able to maintain a lifestyle with so few calories and end up throwing in the towel, thinking losing weight is a feat too big for them.

One thing I realize is that if you're going to go into battle with weight loss, you probably are going to lose. On the other hand, if you have the right approach, it's mapped out and easy to follow, and you're never hungry, then you have a recipe for success. That is exactly what my process is.

My sensible yet scientific three-tier approach is all laid out for you in a simple-to-follow format. Each tier is specifically and scientifically designed to help you conquer certain objectives that will make your weight-loss goal easily achieved. The only thing I need from you is your willingness to commit to following what I have laid out for you, along with your personal desire to reach your goal.

Tier One—Making the Shift

During tier one, your foods and meals will consist of macronutrients and macronutrient divisions that will quickly shift your metabolic rate and jump-start your weight loss. All people, regardless of how much weight they want to drop, will start here. This tier will ensure that your body makes the proper metabolic shift necessary to set you up for successful weight loss while avoiding the all-too-discouraging plateaus usually associated with most diet plans. This will be the strictest part of the process and will last for seven days. This seven-day metabolic-shifting period is designed to accomplish four very important functions:

1. Stabilize blood sugar levels.
2. Stimulate your metabolism.
3. Re-balance your water and electrolytes.
4. Control your cravings.

In this tier, you can expect to lose five to seven pounds as your body goes through this readjustment period. If for any reason you do not see a weight loss of at least five pounds and your cravings are not noticeably more under control, I ask that you stay in tier one until this is accomplished. This will ensure you've have made the proper metabolic shift and your body is running in a much more efficient manner.

There are a few things a small percentage of you may experience during the first three to four days in tier one, including:

» slight shakiness;
» more than normal sweating; and
» headaches.

These are normal reactions. Your body is going through a detox process from something you were never even aware of. You indeed are withdrawing from your sugar addiction. This should be gone by day five.

Once you have reached this point, you will be ready to move into tier two.

Tier Two—Transforming Your Body

Tier two is designed to transform your body through healthy, consistent weight loss. Now that we've weaned you off of your main weight loss stumbling block (sugar), we are ready to adjust your macronutrient divisions. This adjustment will broaden your food base slightly while not disrupting your weight loss but actually helping bring it to a healthy, consistent, manageable level.

This part of the process has ten very important functions that will help get you to your weight-loss goal while keeping your metabolism running at a higher and more efficient rate:

1. Keep your blood sugar levels stabilized
2. Keep your cravings under control
3. Keep your water and electrolyte balance in check
4. Preserve your lean muscle
5. Keep a steady, continued body fat loss
6. Help maintain a feeling of satiety
7. Keep your furnace (metabolism) stoked
8. Retain a higher energy level
9. Better mental focus
10. Noticeably improve your blood chemistry

At this point, you will be noticing some exciting changes taking place and should be feeling much more energetic! There's no assigned time limit to tier two. It will totally depend on the amount of weight you are looking to lose. You should see an *average* weight loss of one to three pounds per week. This is a very healthy weight loss rate and will ensure you are not sacrificing muscle (lean body mass) while dropping undesirable body fat.

Remember (and this is worth repeating): Muscle is calorie active tissue, meaning it is the physical place where calories are burned for energy. This is why it is so critical to have the right macronutrient divisions so we do not sacrifice any lean muscle while losing body fat. We don't want to cripple our fat-burning machine in any way.

Notice how I've highlighted *average*. This is very important to note. Weight loss comes in unpredictable spurts. Everybody is different, and everybody's body will react differently. Some may experience a steady one- or two-pound a week loss while others may lose five pounds one week and zero the next. This is perfectly normal. Your body will go through these adjustment phases as it tries to find its new weight comfort level. Once the adjustments have been made, which is in different increments for each individual, it will allow your weight loss to proceed to its next new comfort level.

The timeline in tier two will depend on each person's individual goal, where he or she is starting from, and his or her desired target weight. For those of you who may not be sure what your healthy body weight range is, there's a standard measuring tool you can find online to help you called a body mass index (BMI) calculator. By using this tool, you can quickly determine where a healthy weight will be according to your gender, age, and height. Your healthy range should fall between 18.5 and 24.9 using this standard measuring tool. Please remember this is only a guideline, and only you will know what a realistic weight-loss goal will be, so set your goal with realistically achievable intentions.

Note: If you are stuck in a weight-loss plateau for over two weeks, I encourage you to go back into the tier one process until your weight loss resumes. This does happen to some individuals, which tells me that your metabolism needs a gentle nudge.

Once you have reached your set target weight, you will be ready to move into tier three.

Tier 3—*the Lifestyle!*

Tier three is where you have reached your desired target weight. This is the point where you will be maintaining your new healthy body weight while continuing to improve your overall health and quality of life. At this point, I encourage you to put the scale back in the closet and let the mirror be your guide. It is now all about the way you look and feel. The food base in tier three will follow similar guidelines as tier two, with again slight adjustments to our macronutrient divisions.

In tier three, you will also have the option to go out one or two times a week and indulge for *one meal that day only* in all the things that have been off limits to you since you began this process, like ice cream, pizza, or even your favorite fast food meal. You can have whatever you desire for one meal that day as long as you return to your newfound lifestyle immediately after. These things will not hurt you if done in moderation. In fact, this can actually nudge your metabolism by shocking your body. You've worked hard, so splurge and enjoy, but go right back to your new eating habits after!

Warning: Splurging and cheat meals may result in a food hangover. A food hangover is very much like an alcohol hangover where you're nauseous and sluggish. Your body will no longer be used to all the processed foods, sugar, and saturated fat and may react to it in a very discomfiting way, as it does to alcohol.

Because of the extraordinary changes you've made with your body, along with the way you feel physically and mentally, it should be an easy decision to make this newfound lifestyle a permanent change in staying lean, healthy, and happy!

Change

Before we move on to my readiness test and then ultimately the process in the following pages, I wanted to give you what I believe are the key ingredients to true, long-lasting change. After reading my self-made acronym, think about the six components it contains when answering the questions on my readiness test. This will be essential to your success, as it will keep you completely honest with your intentions as well as your commitment.

CHANGE

C—Consistency—The key ingredient in making steady and long-lasting change is consistency.

H—Honesty—Being completely honest with yourself about your intentions will be the root of your success.

A—Action—Taking action will put into play the components necessary to make change possible.

N—Necessity—If you necessitate your intentions and actions, they will eventually become newly formed habits.

G—Goals—Set short-, medium-, and long-term goals to help keep you on track in time-lined increments.

E—Enthusiasm—The glue that will hold all of the other components together is enthusiasm; it will make CHANGE enjoyable as well as inevitable.

Readiness Test

So you say you're ready to make your life-changing move. As you've probably noticed throughout the book, I'm a straightforward, completely honest, and direct kind of guy.

That said, the pages of this book are based in fact, not fluff. I am bringing you a simple, proven solution to weight loss that will absolutely work for anyone who is willing to put forth the effort and follow my directions throughout this entire book.

This experience will undoubtedly change your life in an amazing way. However, it will require work on your part. There can be no sort of following this system. You must commit 100 percent to see the results of feeling healthier and looking better. As they say, Rome wasn't built in a day. Your path to healthier living and weight loss is a process—not only because it needs to be done safely but also because it's only effective if you make it a priority.

Before you dive in, I want to make sure you're completely prepared to make the commitment it will take to become another *Get Your Lean On* success story.

The following are a series of questions I've devised. Answer them honestly, and then add up your score at the end of the test. This will be a very good indicator of your success based on willingness, goals and attitude.

Score 1 for not at all, 2 slightly, 3 somewhat, 4 quite, 5 extremely

1. Compared with previous attempts, how motivated to lose weight and regain your health are you?
2. How certain are you that you will stay committed to an outlined system for the time it will take you to reach your goal?

Score 1 for cannot, 2 can somewhat, 3 uncertain, 4 can tolerate well, 5 can easily

3. Consider all outside stress in your life. To what extent can you tolerate the effort required to stick to a process?

Score 1 for unrealistic, 2 somewhat unrealistic, 3 moderately unrealistic, 4 somewhat realistic, 5 very realistic

4. Think honestly about how much weight you hope to lose and how quickly you hope to lose it. Figure a weight loss of one to three pounds per week. How realistic is your expectation?

Score 1 for always, 2 frequently, 3 occasionally, 4 rarely, 5 never

5. While dieting, do you fantasize about eating a lot of your favorite foods?
6. While dieting, do you feel deprived, angry, or upset?

If you scored six to thirteen, it is not a good time for change. Inadequate motivation and commitment and unrealistic goals can get in your way. If you scored fourteen to twenty-one, think about ways to boost your readiness before you begin. If you scored twenty-two to thirty, your path is clear. It is time to take action.

Chapter Five

Making the Shift

Welcome to Tier One

Tier one will consist of macronutrient divisions that will quickly shift your metabolic rate and jump start your weight loss. Everyone, regardless of how much weight he or she wants to drop, will start here. This will ensure that your body makes the proper metabolic shift necessary to set you up for successful weight loss. Tier one will be the strictest part of the process and will last for seven days. During this seven-day metabolic-shifting period, there is absolutely no drinking of any alcoholic beverages; this will hinder the process as well as dehydrate you. This seven-day metabolic shifting period is designed to:

1. Stabilize blood sugar levels
2. Stimulate your metabolism
3. Re-balance your water and electrolytes
4. Control your cravings

In the pages to come, you will see a sample day laid out for you as well as recipes labeled in sections: breakfast, lunch, dinner, and snacks. Pick one meal from each category along with two snacks each day. You will have one serving per meal as well as a snack between meals.

Try to eat approximately every three hours. Along with your meals, as well as throughout the day, you will need to take in a minimum of two quarts of water. This will help flush toxins and fat from your system.

Other allowable beverages are as follows:

Note: **A s**erving equals **eight ounces.**

» water, water, water!
» regular coffees and teas
» decaffeinated coffees and teas
» Crystal Light
» sugar-free Kool-Aid
» vegetable juices (no sugar)
» **c**affeinated diet soda (limit **two** servings a day)

Remember, if for any reason you do not see a weight loss of at least five pounds and your cravings are not noticeably more under control, I ask that you stay in tier one until this is accomplished. This will ensure you have made the proper metabolic shift necessary to move into tier two.

Tier One Sample Day

Let's take a look at a typical day in tier one so you have an understanding of how to structure your meals as well as an idea of the types of foods you will be eating.

Breakfast

Breakfast Sandwich (page 63)

Snack

Peanut Butter and Celery Sticks (page 128)

Lunch

Turkey Pesto Wrap (page 95)

Snack

Nutty Yogurt (page 130)

Dinner

Healthy Beef Stroganoff (page 123)

Tier One Breakfast Recipes

Veggie and Bacon Omelet

- » 1/8 c. onion, chopped
- » 1 small clove garlic, chopped
- » 1/4 c. broccoli florets, chopped
- » 1 oz. organic, low-fat turkey bacon
- » 1 tsp. olive oil
- » 1 c. egg whites
- » 1/2 oz. asiago cheese
- » 1/5 tsp. fresh chives, chopped
- » 1 sprig fresh dill, chopped
- » 1/8 c. cherry tomatoes, diced
- » Salt and pepper

Sauté onion, garlic, broccoli, bacon, and olive oil in nonstick pan over medium-high heat for three minutes. Remove from heat and place in bowl. Pour egg whites into pan, cover, and cook until set. Scatter veggies, bacon and cheese over half of egg, and fold the other half over the top. Slide from pan and top with chives, dill, and tomato and season with salt and pepper.

Serves one. Per Serving: calories 240, fat 10, carbs 5.2, protein 29.6.

Portabella Egg Sandwich

- » 1 portabella mushroom
- » 1 tsp. olive oil
- » Salt and pepper
- » 4 egg whites
- » 1 egg
- » 1 slice Canadian bacon
- » 1 slice medium tomato

Sauté the mushroom in a nonstick pan over medium-high heat in olive oil with salt and pepper until desired doneness. Remove from pan and place on plate. Pour egg whites into pan, cover, and cook until set. Season with salt and pepper, fold into quarters, and place on top of mushroom. Cook remaining whole egg in a pan, flipping when yolk is still soft to make an over-easy egg. Top egg whites with Canadian bacon and tomato, and place over-easy egg on top.

Serves one. Per Serving: calories 241, fat 11.5, carbs 6.5, protein 30.5.

Breakfast Sandwich

» 1 c. egg whites

» 1 slice Canadian bacon

» 1/4 100 percent whole wheat pita pocket

» 1 1/2 tsp. olive oil

Red pepper flakes, onion powder, garlic powder, salt, pepper

Season egg whites with dry seasonings to taste. Cook in nonstick pan over medium heat. Top cooked egg with Canadian bacon. Serve with pita bread, dipped in olive oil.

Serves one. Per Serving: calories 241, fat 9, carbs 5.8, protein 30.2

PB Chocolate Cottage Cheese

- » 2 tsp. unsweetened cocoa
- » Splenda or stevia to taste
- » 2 T. natural peanut butter
- » 1/2 c. low fat cottage cheese
- » 1 tsp. vanilla extract

Mix all ingredients in a bowl and stir well. Microwave a few seconds to warm up if desired.

Serves one. Per Serving: calories 343, fat 17, carbs 15, protein 23.

Mexican Eggs with Almonds

- 1 c. egg whites
- 1/4 c. salsa
- Salt and pepper
- Cilantro
- 15 almonds

Cook egg whites in a nonstick pan over medium heat. Season with salt and pepper. Top egg with salsa and fresh cilantro. Serve with almonds.

Serves one. Per Serving: calories 233, fat 9.2, carbs 7.2, protein 28.7

Scrambled Spinach, Eggs, and Beef

» 1/2 c. egg substitute

» 8 ounces spinach, blanched, drained, and chopped

» 2 T. parmesan cheese

» 1/2 onion, chopped

» 1 T. olive oil

» 1/2 pound lean ground beef

» Add tabasco sauce to taste

Heat oil in a large skillet. Add onion and sauté over medium heat until soft. Add beef and brown. Add in spinach, cooking and stirring for three to four minutes. Mix Tabasco sauce with eggs, and pour over beef mixture. Cook until eggs are set. Remove from heat, and sprinkle with cheese.

Serves three. Per Serving: calories 210, fat 18, carbs 3, protein 16.

Protein Shake

- » 1 heaping scoop 100 percent whey protein powder
- » 1/2 oz. walnuts
- » 1/3 c. fresh raspberries
- » Water

Combine all ingredients in a blender with as much water as desired.

Serves one. Per Serving: calories 252, fat 11, carbs 9, protein 27.5/

Deviled Egg Breakfast

- » 1 T. bread and butter pickle, minced
- » 1 tsp. mustard
- » 1 T. low-fat mayonnaise
- » 6 eggs
- » 1 T. olive oil

Beat eggs, mayo, mustard, and pickles together. Spray heated pan with cooking spray, and add mixture while stirring. Cook until desired consistency.

Serves two. Per Serving: calories 250, fat 22, carbs 1, protein 12

Perfect Soy Pancakes

- 1/4 c. soy protein powder
- 1 T. olive oil
- 1/3 c. low-fat sour cream
- 2 eggs

Mix all ingredients with a whisk. Batter will be runny. Cook on greased skillet as you would regular pancakes. Top with sugar-free syrup or your choice of berries.

Serves one. Per Serving: calories 357, fat 24, carbs 6, protein 27.

Balsamic Egg Salad with Cucumber and Tomato

» 1 hardboiled egg and 5 hardboiled egg whites
» 1/2 c. English cucumber, chopped
» 1/2 c. cherry tomatoes, chopped
» 1 T. balsamic vinegar
» 1 tsp. olive oil
» Salt and pepper

Chop egg and egg whites and combine all ingredients. Season with salt and pepper.

Serves one. Per Serving: calories 226, fat 10.6, carbs 8.5, protein 32.

Cottage Cheese with Cinnamon and Peanut Butter

- 1 c. 1 percent cottage cheese with cinnamon
- 1 T. natural peanut butter

Season cottage cheese with cinnamon. Enjoy peanut butter separately.

Serves one. Per Serving: calories 268, fat 10.3, carbs 9, protein 32.

Italian Omelet

» 1 T. parmesan cheese

» 2 T. low-fat mozzarella cheese, shredded

» 1/4 c. low-fat ricotta cheese

» 1 tsp. Italian seasoning

» 1/2 c. egg substitute

» 1/4 c. diced tomato

Cook eggs as an omelet in a round skillet. Flip eggs once they are almost dry on top. Mix in a bowl ricotta cheese, mozzarella, parmesan, Italian seasoning, and diced tomatoes. Spoon into cooked omelet. Fold in half and place on plate.

Serves one. Per Serving: calories 348, fat 22, carbs 10, protein 27.

Ham and Cheese Scrambled Eggs

- » 1 egg
- » 1/2 c. egg whites
- » 1/4 c. diced ham
- » 1/4 c. reduced-fat cheddar cheese
- » Onion powder, garlic powder, pinch cayenne
- » Green onions, chopped
- » 1/2 slice wheat bread

Beat egg and egg whites in bowl. Add remaining ingredients except green onions and bread. Cook in nonstick pan over medium heat, stirring the entire time, until completely cooked. Garnish with green onions, and serve with dry wheat toast.

Serves one. Per Serving: calories 255.5, fat 9.2, carbs 7.6, protein 32.7.

Mexi Egg Cups

- » 1/2 tsp. pepper
- » 1/4 c. low-fat Monterrey jack cheese
- » Hot pepper sauce to taste
- » 2 oz. green chilies, diced
- » 1.25 c. egg substitute
- » 1/2 c. chicken breast, cooked and chopped

Spray muffin pan with non-stick cooking spray. Preheat oven to 350 degrees. Mix all ingredients together and pour into four muffin cups. Bake for twenty minutes or until set. Cool slightly before serving. Can eat hot or cold.

Serves four. Per Serving: calories 169, fat 9, carbs 4, protein 16.

Quick and Tasty Cottage Cheese

» 1/2 c. cottage cheese

» 1 tsp. Splenda or stevia

» 2 T. chopped almond or walnut

» Cinnamon, to taste

Combine cottage cheese, cinnamon, and Splenda or stevia, and top with almonds.

Serves one. Per Serving: calories 190, fat 11, carbs 8, protein 16.

Tomato Basil Eggs

» 1 tomato, sliced
» 4 fresh basil leaves
» 3 eggs

Beat eggs with fork, and add two minced basil leaves. Spray skillet with cooking spray, and add mixture. Cook until you reach the desired consistency. Place sliced tomato on plate, and top with eggs. Add fresh basil for garnish. Also can be topped with a teaspoon of basil pesto.

Serves one. Per Serving: calories 243, fat 15, carbs 7, protein 20.

Zucchini Frittata

- » 1/4 c. parmesan cheese
- » 1/2 tsp. oregano
- » 1 T. olive oil
- » 1 medium tomato, seeded and chopped
- » 1 medium zucchini, thinly sliced
- » 1 c. low-fat cottage cheese
- » 6 eggs
- » 1 tsp. dried basil

Beat eggs in a bowl with basil and oregano. Stir in cottage cheese and half of the parmesan. In a large skillet, add oil and sauté tomato and zucchini until zucchini is lightly browned. Pour in the egg mixture, and sprinkle with remaining cheese. Cook over medium-low heat until eggs are set, about fifteen minutes. Cut into wedges and serve.

Serves four. Per Serving: calories 231, fat 14, carbs 6, protein 20.

Finally...Cereal

- » 1/2 c. textured vegetable protein, tvp
- » 1 T. sugar-free maple syrup, optional
- » Stevia or Splenda to taste
- » 2 tsp. Smart Balance butter
- » 1 tsp. cinnamon, optional
- » 1 c. unsweetened soymilk

Place tvp and soymilk in a microwave-safe bowl and cook for three minutes on high. Cover with plastic wrap and let sit ten minutes. Add more soymilk if needed. Add optional other ingredients and Smart Balance butter and enjoy your cereal at last!

Serves one. Per Serving: calories 305, fat 8, carbs 18, protein 35.

Canadian Bacon and Cabbage Hash Browns

» 2 T. onion, chopped

» 1 count egg

» 1 T. canola oil

» 4 slices Canadian bacon

» 2 c. cabbage, thinly sliced

Combine cabbage, onion, and egg in a bowl. Stir until well combined. Heat canola oil in a skillet over medium-high heat. With hands, clump the mixture and form into two patties. Place the patties in a skillet and brown on both sides. Serve one hash brown with two slices of Canadian bacon. Enjoy! Can also be served with two scrambled or over-easy eggs if desired.

Serves two. Per Serving: calories 205, fat 13, carbs 5, protein 16.

Asparagus Frittata

- 1/2 c. reduced-fat cheese
- 1/2 lb. asparagus spear, trimmed and cut into half-inch pieces
- 1 T. olive oil
- 6 eggs

Preheat oven to 350 degrees. Boil water in a skillet, and cook asparagus until it is crisp and tender. Drain and plunge into ice water to stop cooking. Coat oven-proof skillet with olive oil, and heat over medium heat. Mix eggs, cheese, and asparagus in a bowl. Add eggs to skillet. Cook over medium heat until bottom is set and then transfer skillet to oven and bake until top is set. Serve warm or at room temperature.

Serves two. Per Serving: calories 344, fat 24, carbs 4, protein 27.

Tier One Lunch Recipes

Chicken with Corn and Avocado

- » 20 oz. chicken breast
- » 1 c. corn
- » 1/2 avocado
- » 2 tsp. olive oil
- » 1 tsp. ground cumin
- » Hot sauce
- » Salt and pepper

Cook chicken breast in a nonstick pan over medium heat. Season chicken with hot sauce, salt, pepper, and cumin. When juices run clear, remove chicken from pan. Top each five-ounce serving with 1/4 c. corn, 1/8 of the avocado, and a 1/2 tsp. olive oil.

Serves four. Per Serving: calories 258, fat 9.5, carbs 9, protein 34.

Tuna Salad

- » 12 oz. canned tuna in water, drained and pressed
- » 1/4 c. Dijon mustard
- » 1/4 c. plain, nonfat Greek yogurt
- » 1 c. chopped celery
- » 4 slices Canadian bacon, chopped
- » 1 tsp. fresh basil, chopped
- » 1 tsp. red pepper flakes
- » Salt and pepper
- » 1 avocado, sliced

Combine all ingredients except avocado. Top each serving with 1/4 of the avocado.

Serves four. Per Serving: calories 261, fat 9.3, carbs 7, protein 33.

Egg Salad

- 4 hardboiled eggs and 20 hardboiled egg whites
- 1/4 T. Dijon mustard
- 1 c. celery, chopped
- 1 c. green pepper, chopped
- 1 c. plain, nonfat Greek yogurt
- 1/4 c. mayo with olive oil
- 3 T. fresh lemon juice
- 3 T. chives, chopped
- Salt and pepper

Chop egg and egg whites, and combine all ingredients.

Serves four. Per Serving: calories 244, fat 9, carbs 7, protein 31.

Curry Salad with Grilled Shrimp

- 1 tsp. Splenda or stevia
- 1/4 c. olive oil
- 4 c. mixed lettuce
- 1/2 lemon, juiced
- 1 lemon wedge
- 16 jumbo shrimp
- 1 T. hot pepper sauce
- 1 1/2 tsp. curry powder

Skewer shrimp with four wooden skewers. Stir together oil, curry powder, Splenda or stevia, lemon juice, and pepper sauce. Place shrimp in a pan and cover with dressing. Grill shrimp for sixty seconds per side or until pink. Place shrimp on greens, and squeeze lemon juice over salad.

Serves four. Per Serving: calories 259, fat 16, carbs 5, protein 25.

Veggie Shrimp Patties

» 1 tsp. sesame oil
» 1/4 c. onion, chopped
» 1 T. light soy sauce
» 1 tsp. garlic powder
» 6 eggs
» 4 T. canola oil
» 2 c. cabbage, shredded
» 1/4 tsp. black pepper
» 1 c. bean sprouts
» 1 c. tiny cocktail shrimp, cooked

Add two tablespoons olive oil to pan and sauté onions and cabbage until tender over medium-high heat. Remove and drain excess liquid. Whisk eggs in a bowl. Mix in light soy sauce, spices, sesame oil, sprouts, and onion and cabbage mixture. Heat remaining olive oil in a skillet and ladle four ounces of mixture into the pan. Sprinkle tops with shrimp. Cook about three minutes or until edges begin to brown. Flip over and cook another three to four minutes. Enjoy.

Serves two. Per Serving: calories 560, fat 38, carbs 13, protein 44.

Avocado Tuna Salad

- » 1/2 c. red onion, chopped
- » 1 c. mashed avocado
- » 2 T. light mayonnaise
- » 2 tsp. hot pepper sauce
- » 1 fresh lemon, juiced
- » 2 eggs, hard boiled
- » 2 count dill pickle, chopped
- » 1 6-oz. can tuna in water, drained

Peel eggs and mash with a fork. Peel avocados and mash, adding lemon juice. Drain water from tuna and mix with onions, eggs, avocados, pickles, pepper sauce, and light mayo. Serve over lettuce.

Serves two. Per Serving: calories 339, fat 20, carbs 12, protein 28.

Tuna on the Go

» 2 T. low fat Monterrey jack cheese, shredded
» 1 1/2 c. frozen broccoli floret, chopped
» 1/2 c. cottage cheese, 2 percent fat
» 3 oz. tuna, water packed and drained

Place all ingredients in a microwave-safe dish and microwave it for two minutes.

Serves one. Per Serving: calories 237, fat 5, carbs 12, protein 36.

Dijon Chicken and Broccoli

» 1/2 c. reduced-sodium chicken broth

» 1 T. olive oil

» 3 T. Dijon mustard

» 1 garlic clove, minced

» 1/2 tsp. ground ginger

» 1 1/2 T. light soy sauce

» 1 lb. chicken breast, thinly sliced

» 4 c. broccoli florets

Mix chicken broth and soy sauce and then set aside. Cook broccoli and garlic in hot oil in a large pan at medium-high heat until crisp tender. Remove and keep warm. Add chicken to pan and cook through. Add broth mixture, and bring to a boil. Reduce heat to medium-low and stir in mustard and ginger. Return broccoli to pan and toss to coat until heated through. Serve over cabbage rice if desired.

Serves four. Per Serving: calories 228, fat 12, carbs 6, protein 23.

Turkey Burger with Portabella Bun

» 16 oz. 93 percent lean ground turkey
» 4 oz. reduced-fat feta cheese
» 1 c. red onion, chopped
» 2 cloves garlic, chopped
» 2 tsp. cumin
» 2 tsp. chili powder
» 1 c. fresh spinach
» 4 portabella mushrooms
» Salt and pepper

Combine all ingredients except spinach and mushrooms. Form into patties. Remove gills from mushrooms with spoon. Season with salt and pepper. Grill burgers and mushrooms until desired wellness. Serve burgers over mushrooms, topped with spinach.

Serves four. Per Serving: calories 250, fat 11, carbs 8, protein 30.

Asian Beef Lettuce Wrap

- » 1 8-oz. can water chestnuts, finely chopped
- » 2 tsp. sesame oil
- » 1 T. rice wine vinegar
- » 1 T. pickled ginger, minced
- » 1 T. olive oil
- » 1 medium onion, chopped
- » 1 T. light soy sauce
- » 1 lb. lean ground beef
- » 16 count large lettuce leaf
- » 1/4 c. hoisin sauce
- » 1 green onion, chopped
- » 2 cloves of garlic, chopped
- » 1 tsp. Asian chili sauce

In a medium skillet over medium-high heat, brown ground beef in one tablespoon of oil. Drain and set aside. Cook onion in the same pan and add garlic until softened. Stir in soy sauce, hoisin, ginger, vinegar, and chili sauce. Then add green onion, water chestnuts, and sesame oil. Cook for about two minutes. Serve mixture in lettuce leaves, and wrap like a taco.

Serves four. Per Serving: calories 377, fat 26, carbs 13, protein 23.

Lemon Haddock with Capers and Prosciutto

- 12 oz. haddock
- 1 lemon, juiced
- 1/4 c. capers
- 1 clove garlic, pressed
- 1 c. mushrooms, sliced
- 2 oz. prosciutto, chopped

Preheat oven to 375 degrees. Place haddock in nine-by-eleven-inch baking dish. Squeeze lemon juice over fish. Scatter capers, garlic, mushrooms, and prosciutto over fish. Bake uncovered for thirty minutes.

Serves four. Per Serving: calories 253, fat 11, carbs 6.5, protein 33.

Vegetarian Spinach Casserole

» 1 c. reduced-fat cheddar cheese
» Pepper to taste
» 2 tsp. lemon juice
» 1 c. low-fat cottage cheese
» 2 tsp. onion powder
» 2 T. parmesan cheese, grated
» 7 eggs
» 8 c. fresh baby spinach, cooked and drained
» 2 tsp. dried basil
» 1 c. cooked brown rice
» 1/2 tsp. cayenne pepper

Preheat oven to 350 degrees. Mix three eggs, lemon juice, brown rice, dried basil, parmesan, and onion powder together for layer one. In a separate bowl mix spinach, cottage cheese, cheddar cheese, four eggs, cayenne pepper, and pepper together for layer two. Spread the first-layer ingredients in the bottom of a greased casserole dish. Spread the second-layer ingredients over the top. Bake for forty-five to sixty minutes.

Serves four. Per Serving: calories 153, fat 5, carbs 8, protein 19.

Sautéed Balsamic Shrimp with Vegetables and Bacon

- » 16 oz. raw shrimp
- » 1 c. cherry tomatoes, diced
- » 1 c. mushrooms, sliced
- » 1 c. yellow peppers, chopped
- » 8 oz. organic, low-fat turkey bacon, diced
- » 2 1/2 T. olive oil
- » 1/4 c. balsamic vinegar

Sauté all ingredients in a nonstick pan, over medium-high heat for about seven minutes or until shrimp are no longer translucent.

Serves four. Per Serving: calories 247.5, fat 11, carbs 7, protein 28.5.

Turkey Pesto Wrap

» 2 oz. sliced turkey breast
» 1/4 red onion, thinly sliced
» 1/4 c. red bell pepper, thinly sliced
» 2 large lettuce leaves
» 2 T. black olive, sliced
» 1 T. basil pesto

Lay lettuce leaves flat on plate. Place turkey on leaves. Top with peppers, onion, black olives, and pesto sauce. Roll up and enjoy!

Serves one. Per Serving: calories 169, fat 10, carbs 8, protein 13.

New Orleans Chicken

- » 2 1/2 oz. chicken breast, cut in chunks
- » 1 smart chicken Andouille sausage
- » 1/4 c. zucchini, sliced
- » 1/4 c. red pepper, chopped
- » 1/8 c. onion, chopped
- » 1 bay leaf
- » 1 clove garlic, chopped
- » 1/2 tsp. fresh thyme
- » 1/2 T. fresh parsley
- » Pinch cayenne
- » Salt and pepper

Sauté all ingredients in a nonstick pan over medium-high heat until juices of chicken run clear.

Serves four. Per Serving: calories 250, fat 10, carbs 7.9, protein 32.

Greek Turkey Breasts

- 20 oz. turkey breast meat
- 1 clove garlic
- 3/4 c. cherry tomatoes, diced
- 24 black olives, sliced
- 4 oz. reduced fat feta cheese
- 1/4 c. capers
- 1 lemon, juiced

Brown turkey breast, garlic, and tomatoes in a nonstick pan over medium heat. Remove turkey breasts from pan and place on plate. Pour tomatoes over turkey. Top with remaining ingredients and fresh lemon juice.

Serves four. Per Serving: calories 248, fat 9.5, carbs 10, protein 30.

Oriental Lettuce Wraps

» 1 tsp. sambal oelek (or more)

» 1 T. reduced-sodium soy sauce

» 1/2 c. red bell pepper, chopped

» Parmesan cheese (optional)

» 1 T. oyster sauce

» 1 onion, chopped

» 1 lb. lean ground beef

» 1 T. garlic

» 1/4 c. cucumber, peeled, seeded, and chopped

» 4 to 6 crisp lettuce leafs

Spray skillet with nonstick spray and add ground beef, onion, and garlic. Cook until beef is almost cooked through, about five to six minutes. Add cucumber and red pepper and cook for five minutes. Add soy sauce, oyster sauce, and sambal oelek. Mix well and reduce mixture to about half. Place two tablespoons of mixture on a lettuce leaf, roll, and serve. Sprinkle with parmesan cheese if desired.

Serves four. Per Serving: calories 290, fat 19, carbs 5, protein 22.

Tasty Tuna Salad

- 1 6-oz. can tuna in water, drained
- 1 c. low-fat cottage cheese
- 1/4 c. low-fat mayonnaise
- 1 tsp. lemon pepper seasoning
- 1 tsp. lemon juice
- 1/4 c. green onion, chopped
- 2 T. fresh parsley, chopped
- 3 eggs
- 1/4 c. celery, chopped
- 1/4 tsp. celery salt

Place eggs in saucepan and cover with cold water. Bring to a boil, cover, and remove from heat. Let eggs sit in hot water for ten to twelve minutes. Remove, let cool, and chop. In a large bowl, flake tuna. Add cottage cheese, eggs, onions, parsley, lemon pepper, celery salt, lemon juice, and mayo. Mix well and chill. Serve in lettuce leaf as a wrap or over mixed greens.

Serves four. Per Serving: calories 290, fat 9, carbs 5, protein 43.

Cilantro Chicken Salad with Peanut Dressing

» 2 tsp. sesame oil

» 1/4 c. rice vinegar

» 2 tsp. peanut oil

» 1/4 c. natural peanut butter, creamy

» 8 c. mixed lettuce

» 1 lime, juiced

» 1 1/2 T. light soy sauce

» 1 T. honey

» 1 garlic clove, minced

» 1 T. fresh ginger, minced

» 1/4 c. fresh cilantro, chopped

» 1 tsp. chili powder

» 4 chicken breasts, grilled

In a blender, puree oils, peanut butter, vinegar, lime juice, soy sauce, honey, garlic, ginger, and chili powder. Slice chicken breast, and toss lettuce with dressing.

Serves four. Per Serving: calories 242, fat 6, carbs 17, protein 31.

Chicken and Walnut Salad

- 1/4 c. walnut, chopped
- 1 bag mixed salad green
- 3 T. extra-virgin olive oil
- 1 tsp. dried basil
- 2 cooked chicken breasts
- 3 T. balsamic vinegar

In a saucepan, combine olive oil, balsamic vinegar, basil, and walnuts. Cook until somewhat thickened and liquid is reduced. Place greens on salad dish, and place chicken on top. Drizzle with dressing.

Serves two. Per Serving: calories 410, fat 31, carbs 4, protein 31.

Tier One Dinners

Spicy Hot Turkey

- » 12 oz. turkey tenderloin
- » Pickle juice
- » Jalapeno
- » 1 c. plain nonfat Greek yogurt
- » 1/4 c. Dijon mustard
- » Salt and pepper
- » 4 c. snap peas
- » 1 1/2 T. olive oil

Place tenderloin in slow cooker. Cover with pickle juice. Cut a slit in the jalapeno with a knife and drop it into the juice. Cook tenderloin for five to seven hours on high. Remove tenderloin from low cooker and shred. Mix in yogurt, mustard, salt and pepper.

Steam pea pods for five minutes. Drizzle with olive oil and season with salt and pepper.

Serves three. Per Serving: calories 231, fat 9, carbs 7, protein 29.

Salmon with Asparagus

- » 14 oz. salmon
- » 1 lemon, juiced
- » 2 T. Dijon mustard
- » 24 spears asparagus
- » 1/2 c. onion, chopped
- » 1 c. mushrooms, chopped
- » 1 c. celery, chopped
- » 2 T. fresh chives, chopped
- » 2 T. fresh basil, chopped
- » 1 tsp. ground fennel
- » Salt and pepper

Place salmon fillets in nine-by-eleven baking dish. Whisk together lemon juice and mustard. Pour over fish. Lay asparagus spears on all four sides of the fish. Scatter chopped vegetables and herbs over fish and asparagus. Sprinkle with ground fennel, salt, and pepper. Bake, uncovered, for twenty-five to thirty minutes at 375 degrees.

Serves four. Per Serving: calories 242, fat 8.7, carbs 8, protein 28.5.

BBQ Chicken and Garlic Broccoli

- » 16 oz. chicken breast
- » 1/2 c. BBQ sauce
- » 4 c. chopped broccoli
- » 1 lemon, juiced
- » 3 cloves garlic, pressed/minced
- » 1 1/2 T. olive oil
- » Red pepper flakes
- » Salt and pepper

Place chicken breasts in a nine-by-eleven-inch baking dish. Spread BBQ sauce over chicken. Sprinkle red pepper flakes over BBQ sauce. Bake, covered, for twenty-five minutes at 350 degrees. Sauté broccoli, garlic, olive oil, a tsp. of red pepper flakes, salt, and pepper for five to seven minutes.

Serves four. Per Serving: calories 224, fat 8, carbs 8.6, protein 29.

Grilled Tenderloin with Tangy Onion Salad

- 1/2 c. low-carb French salad dressing
- 1 large red onion, thinly sliced
- 2 T. caper
- 1.25 lb. beef tenderloin steak
- 1 4-oz. can black olives, sliced
- 1 bag romaine lettuce, chopped

Grill or broil tenderloin and let rest ten minutes before slicing. Placed sliced tenderloin in a bowl with the dressing, onions, capers, and olives. Toss to coat. Place mixture over salad greens.

Serves four. Per Serving: calories 397, fat 22, carbs 7, protein 36.

Turkey Green Chili

» 4 oz. low-fat turkey sausage, casing removed
» 2 lb. turkey breast tenderloin, cubed
» 6 oz. tomatillo, husked and chopped
» 12 oz. poblano chili
» 1 1/2 c. onion, chopped
» 1 T. olive oil
» 1 T. lime juice
» 1 c. low-sodium chicken broth
» 1/2 c. jalapeno chili, chopped
» 1 1/2 tsp. cumin
» 1/4 c. cilantro, chopped
» 3 cloves of garlic, chopped
» 1 1/2 T. chili powder
» 1/2 c. canned tomato, diced

Char poblanos under broiler until all sides are blackened. Enclose in paper bag; let stand for ten minutes. Peel, seed, and chop. Heat oil in a large pot and add sausage. Sauté until cooked through. Add onions and garlic. Cover and cook ten minutes. Mix in seasonings, and then add turkey breast to pot and stir. Add broth, tomatillos, canned tomatoes, cilantro, lime juice, and jalapeño chilis. Mix in roasted poblanos. Bring to a boil; reduce to medium-low heat. Simmer until turkey is tender, about forty-five minutes. Season with more lime juice if needed.

Serves eight. Per Serving: calories 283, fat 13, carbs 11, protein 30.

Pancetta-Stuffed Chicken Breast with Peas

» 12 oz. chicken breast
» 1 light string cheese
» 4 oz. pancetta
» 1 1/2 c. frozen peas
» Garlic powder
» Salt and pepper
» Fresh parsley, chopped

Pound four 3-oz. chicken breasts until thin enough to stuff and fold over. Shred string cheese and divide it among chicken breasts. Place one ounce of pancetta onto each chicken breast. Roll chicken and place seam down in nine-by-eleven-inch baking dish. Pour peas into pan. Season everything with garlic powder, salt, and pepper. Garnish with fresh parsley.

Serves four. Per Serving: calories 256, fat 11, carbs 7.5, protein 29.7.

Halibut with Spinach and Artichokes

- 16 oz. halibut
- 1 lemon, juiced
- 1/4 c. balsamic vinegar
- 2 T. olive oil
- 4 oz. canned artichokes, quartered
- 2 T. shallot, chopped
- 2 cloves garlic, chopped
- 2 T. fresh basil, chopped
- Salt and pepper
- 1/2 tsp. cayenne
- 1/2 tsp. ground fennel
- 1/2 tsp. thyme
- 4 c. fresh spinach

Place halibut fillets in nine-by-eleven-inch baking dish. Whisk together lemon juice, balsamic vinegar, and olive oil and pour over fish. Rinse artichokes with cold water and drain. Disperse artichokes, shallot, garlic, and basil over fish. Season with dry seasonings. Bake, uncovered, for twenty-five to thirty minutes at 375 degrees. Serve over fresh spinach.

Serves four. Per Serving: calories 252.9, fat 10.4, carbs 7.7, protein 32.2.

Salmon with Soy and Broccoli

- 16 oz. salmon
- 2 c. broccoli, chopped
- 1/4 c. soy sauce
- 1 lemon, juiced
- Salt and pepper
- 2 cloves garlic, pressed
- 2 tsp. fresh mint, chopped
- 1/4 c. organic bread crumbs

Place salmon fillets in nine-by-eleven-inch baking dish. Disperse broccoli around fish. Pour soy sauce over fish and broccoli. Squeeze lemon over fish and broccoli. Season with salt and pepper. Scatter garlic and mint over fillets and broccoli. Sprinkle fish with bread crumbs. Bake, uncovered, for twenty-five to thirty minutes at 375 degrees.

Serves four. Per Serving: calories 276, fat 10, carbs 8.7, protein 32.2

Shrimp Guacamole

- » 20 oz. raw shrimp
- » 2–3 limes, juiced (about 2 fl. oz.)
- » 2 tsp. olive oil
- » 1 avocado, diced
- » 1/2 c. red onion, diced
- » 1 clove garlic, chopped
- » 1 jalapeno, diced
- » 2 T. fresh cilantro, chopped
- » Salt and pepper

Sauté shrimp in lime juice and olive oil in a nonstick pan over medium-high heat for about seven minutes or until shrimp are no longer translucent. Remove from heat and pour into bowl. You may cut the shrimp into thirds if you prefer. Combine all remaining ingredients.

Serves four. Per Serving: calories 244.8, fat 10.5, carbs 7, protein 30.8.

Mexican Ground Turkey

- 16 oz. extra-lean ground turkey
- 1/2 c. diced green chilies
- 2 cloves garlic, chopped
- 1/2 c. red onion, diced
- 2 1/2 T. olive oil
- 1 c. cherry tomatoes, halved
- 1/2 c. corn
- 1/2 c. mushrooms, diced
- Salt and pepper
- 2 tsp. ground cumin
- 1 tsp. chili powder
- 1/2 tsp. oregano
- 1 pinch red pepper flakes
- 1 T. fresh cilantro, chopped

Brown turkey, chilies, garlic, and red onion with olive oil in a nonstick pan, over medium heat. Add tomatoes, corn, mushrooms, and dry seasonings and cook for an additional three to five minutes. Garnish with fresh cilantro.

Serves four. Per Serving: calories 252.9, fat 10.4, carbs 7.7, protein 32.2.

Swordfish with Spicy Tomato Salsa

- » 4 6-oz. swordfish steaks
- » 1/2 c. red onion, chopped
- » 4 plum tomato, seeded and chopped
- » 1/4 c. olive oil
- » 4 T. olive oil
- » 1 bag mixed greens
- » 2 T. lemon juice
- » 12 oz. green beans, cooked until crisp tender
- » 1/2 cucumber, peeled, seeded, and diced
- » 1 clove of garlic, chopped
- » 1/2 c. cilantro, chopped
- » 2 T. balsamic vinegar
- » 1/2 tsp. cayenne pepper
- » Pepper to taste

Make salad dressing by adding 1/4 c. olive oil to two tablespoons lemon juice. Make salsa by adding plum tomatoes, red onions, garlic, cilantro, balsamic vinegar, two tablespoons olive oil, cayenne pepper, and cucumber together. Rub swordfish with two tablespoons olive oil and pepper. Place fish on preheated grill at medium flame, and cook each side for two to four minutes. Add dressing to salad greens and beans. Place fish on top of greens, and spoon tomato salsa on top.

Serves four. Per Serving: calories 524, fat 35, carbs 17, protein 38.

Spaghetti Squash and Turkey Casserole

- 2 1/4 c. reduced-fat sharp cheddar cheese
- 1/4 c. red onion, diced
- 1 red bell pepper, diced
- 1/4 tsp. pepper
- 1 lb. ground turkey breast
- 2 garlic cloves, minced
- 1 tsp. dried oregano
- 2 tsp. dried basil
- 1 spaghetti squash, halved and seeded
- 1 14.5-oz can of Italian-style diced tomatoes

Preheat oven to 375 degrees. Place squash on a baking sheet and bake for forty minutes or until tender. Remove from heat, cool, and shred pulp with a fork. Reduce oven temp to 350 degrees. Spray nonstick spray on a casserole dish. In a skillet over medium heat, brown turkey and mix in red pepper, onion, and garlic. Cook until veggies are tender. Mix shredded squash and tomatoes in skillet, and add seasonings. Cook until heated through. Remove skillet from heat and add two cups of cheese until melted. Transfer to casserole dish. Bake for twenty-five minutes and then sprinkle with remaining cheese. Bake for an additional five minutes until cheese is melted.

Serves four. Per Serving: calories 306, fat 13, carbs 9, protein 40.

Chicken Breast and Red Pepper Soup with Cheesy Broiled Bell Peppers

» 2 T. black olives, chopped

» 1 c. bottled roasted red sweet pepper, drained and chopped

» 1/2 red bell pepper, seeded and cut into strips

» 1/4 tsp. pepper

» 1/2 c. onion, chopped

» 2 medium zucchini, halved and sliced 1/4-inch thick

» 3/4 c. low fat Monterrey jack cheese, shredded

» 1/2 green bell pepper, seeded and cut into strips

» 2 tsp. garlic powder

» 1 tsp. dried oregano

» 4 chicken breasts

» 2 tsp. dried basil

» 1/4 tsp. cayenne pepper

» 2 T. balsamic vinegar

» 1 14.5-oz can diced tomatoes

» 2 14.5-oz can low-sodium chicken broth

» 2 c. steamed crisp tender green beans, chopped

» 1/2 yellow bell pepper, seeded and cut into strips

Chicken Breast and Red Pepper Soup

Slice chicken breasts into one-inch pieces. In a slow cooker, combine chicken with chicken broth, diced tomatoes, basil, oregano, garlic powder, roasted red peppers, onion, balsamic vinegar, and pepper. Cover and cook six to eight hours on low heat or three to four hours on high heat. Add zucchini and beans and cook on high for twenty minutes or until crisp tender.

Cheesy Broiled Bell Peppers

Arrange peppers on ungreased broiler pie pan nine by two inches. Sprinkle with cheese, olives, and cayenne. Set oven to broil. Broil three to four inches from heat for about three to five minutes, until cheese is melted.

Serves four. Per Serving: calories 291, fat 5, carbs 19, protein 43.

Southwestern Grilled Pork Tenderloin with Roasted Cauliflower

» 2 tsp. fresh rosemary

» 1/8 tsp. garlic powder

» 3/4 tsp. ground cumin

» 1 T. olive oil

» 1 1/2 lb. pork tenderloin

» 1 small head cauliflower, cut into 1-inch florets

» 1 1/2 tsp. dried oregano

» 1 tsp. fresh garlic, chopped

» 4 tsp. chili powder

Southwestern Grilled Pork Tenderloin

Mix chili powder, dried oregano, ground cumin, and garlic powder together. Place tenderloins on a plate, and rub the dry mixture over the pork. Cover and refrigerate for six to twenty-four hours. Grill pork over medium coals or broil for approximately twenty-five to thirty minutes.

Roasted Cauliflower

In a bowl, toss cauliflower with oil, rosemary, and garlic. Arrange on a baking pan and roast in oven at 450 degrees for approximately thirty minutes or until brown and tender.

Serves four. Per Serving: calories 253, fat 9, carbs 4, protein 37.

Mediterranean Chicken and Soy Beans

- » 1 tsp. white wine vinegar
- » 2 tomatoes, chopped
- » 1 tsp. red wine vinegar
- » 8 pitted kalamata olive, halved
- » 1/2 onion, chopped
- » 2 T. olive oil
- » 1 T. garlic clove, minced
- » 1/4 c. fresh herb of choice, chopped - yes this is correct.
- » 1 fresh basil leaf, chopped
- » 2 chicken breasts, bone in
- » 1 15-oz. can soybeans

Preheat oven to 375 degrees. Place each chicken breast on a large square of aluminum foil. Combine one of the chopped tomatoes, onion, olives, one tablespoon olive oil, white wine vinegar, and basil; spoon over chicken. Fold foil up and seal to form a packet. Bake until chicken is cooked through, about twenty to thirty minutes.

For the beans, heat saucepan over medium heat and add one tablespoon olive oil. Add garlic and cook for two minutes. Add soybeans, chopped tomato, herbs, and red wine vinegar and cook for five minutes until heated through. Carefully open chicken packets and transfer to two plates. Serve beans alongside chicken.

Serves four. Per Serving: calories 253, fat 9, carbs 4, protein 37.

Chipotle Turkey Meatloaf and Cauliflower Mashed Potatoes

» 1/4 c. wheat bran
» 1/4 c. sour cream, light
» 2 T. Smart Balance butter, melted
» 1 tsp. salt substitute
» 1 tsp. onion powder
» 2 Italian turkey sausage, casing removed
» 1 lb. ground turkey breast
» 2 T. garlic, chopped
» 1/4 c. flaxseed, ground
» 1 c. enchilada sauce
» 2 tsp. cumin
» 1 egg
» 2 chipotle chilies in adobo
» 1 cauliflower, whole head
» 1 4-oz. can green chilies, diced

Turkey Meatloaf

Preheat oven to 350. In a large bowl, combine turkey breast, sausage, egg, flaxseed, wheat bran, green chilies, chopped chipotle chilies, one tablespoon garlic, cumin, onion powder, and 1/4 cup enchilada sauce. Mix well. Place in a bread pan or nine-by-thirteen casserole dish, cover with remaining 3/4 cup enchilada sauce, and bake approximately forty to forty-five minutes.

Cauliflower Mashed Potatoes

Break cauliflower into florets and steam until tender. Place in a blender or food processor and puree. Add butter, remaining tablespoon of garlic, sour cream, and salt substitute. Blend well. Serve with extra smart balance or sour cream. (Low-fat cheese is excellent too!)

Serves four. Per Serving: calories 439, fat 25, carbs 19, protein 39.

Sun-Dried Tomato–Stuffed Chicken with Greek Artichoke Salad

» 2 12-oz. can artichoke hearts, drained and chopped

» 1/2 c. spinach, fresh and torn

» 2 roma tomatoes, chopped

» 4 oz. reduced-fat feta cheese

» 1/2 red onion, thinly sliced

» 1/4 c. parmesan cheese

» 3 T. garlic, minced

» 2 T. fresh spearmint leaves, chopped

» 1/4 c. fresh lemon juice

» 2 T. extra-virgin olive oil

» 1 cucumber, peeled, seeded, and chopped

» 6 chicken breasts pounded to 1/4-inch thickness

» 1/2 c. basil, fresh and chopped

» 1 4-oz. can black olives, sliced

» 3 oz. sun-dried tomatoes, hydrated and chopped

Sun-Dried Tomato–Stuffed Chicken

Combine in a bowl sun-dried tomatoes, parmesan cheese, 1/4 cup basil, 2 T. garlic, 2 T. lemon juice, and spinach. Take pounded chicken breasts and place two to three tablespoons of filling in each. Roll up and secure with a toothpick. Bake at 350 for twenty to twenty-five minutes or until no longer pink. (Can also grill, which is fabulous.)

Greek Salad

In a large bowl, combine artichoke hearts, roma tomatoes (seeded preferred), red onion, drained black olives, one tablespoon garlic, cucumber, feta, 1/4 cup basil, spearmint, olive oil, and two tablespoons fresh lemon juice. Mix well and let rest at least thirty minutes.

Serves six. Per Serving: calories 447, fat 23, carbs 28, protein 32.

Healthy Beef Stroganoff

» 1/2 c. onion, diced

» 1/2 c. mushrooms, sliced

» 1/2 c. low-fat mayonnaise

» 1/2 c. low-sodium beef bouillon

» 1/2 c. low-fat sour cream

» 1 lb. lean ground beef

» 1 tsp. garlic powder

» 1 tsp. dry mustard

» 4 zucchinis

Sauté onions and mushrooms in a nonstick pan coated with cooking spray. When tender, add ground beef and cook until no longer pink. Combine sour cream, mayo, seasonings, and bouillon. Blend into meat mixture and cook fifteen minutes over low heat.

For zucchini noodles, take a potato peeler and peel zucchini into ribbon-like pieces. Sauté over medium heat in a little olive oil until tender or steam. Serve beef mixture over zucchini noodles. Enjoy!

Serves four. Per Serving: calories 357, fat 19, carbs 15, protein 30.

Tuna Steaks with Artichoke Salsa

- » 2 roma tomatoes, chopped
- » 1/2 c. red onion, thinly sliced
- » 1/4 c. parmesan cheese, grated
- » 2 T. olive oil
- » 1 lemon, juiced
- » 2 tsp. dried basil
- » 1 cucumber, peeled, seeded, and chopped
- » 1 4-oz. can black olives, sliced
- » 1 12-oz. can artichoke hearts, drained and chopped
- » 4 6-oz. tuna steaks

Grill tuna steaks until desired doneness—about five to eight minutes per side for medium rare to medium steaks. (Can use any fish desired.) Combine the rest of the salsa ingredients in a medium bowl, and serve over the top of each steak. Yum!

Serves four. Per Serving: calories 422, fat 20, carbs 16, protein 46.

Grilled Asian Pork Tenderloin with Asian Cucumber Salad

- 1 T. pickled ginger
- 1 1/2 lb. pork tenderloin
- 1 tsp. Splenda or stevia
- 1 tsp. sesame oil
- 1 tsp. prepared horseradish
- 2 T. peanuts, finely chopped
- 1/2 tsp. onion powder
- 1 tsp. minced garlic
- 1 minced garlic clove
- 2 T. light soy sauce
- 1/2 c. light soy sauce
- 1/2 large red onion, thinly sliced
- 2 tsp. hot Chinese mustard
- 1 tsp. ginger, chopped
- 2 cucumbers, peeled, seeded, and thinly sliced
- 1 c. cornstarch
- 1/2 c. cooking sherry
- 1/2 tsp. chili paste
- 1 T. rice wine vinegar
- 1 avocado, peeled, pitted, and sliced
- Pepper to taste

Grilled Asian Pork Tenderloin

Combine 1/2 cup soy sauce, sherry, mustard, horseradish, one clove minced garlic, ginger, red pepper, and onion powder. Pour into a Ziploc bag and add pork. Refrigerate overnight. Heat grill to medium-high. Remove pork from marinade and reserve the marinade. Grill pork twenty-five to thirty minutes or until done. While pork is grilling, cook marinade on stove until boiling. Add a little water to cornstarch and add slowly to boiling marinade to thicken. When tenderloin is done, thinly slice and top with sauce.

Asian Cucumber Salad

For the dressing, mix two tablespoons soy sauce, pickled ginger, sesame oil, rice wine vinegar, chili paste, Splenda, one teaspoon minced garlic, and pepper together. Refrigerate for several hours to blend together flavors. Place cucumber, red onion, and avocado in a bowl. Add dressing and mix well.

Serves four. Per Serving: calories 428, fat 17, carbs 17, protein 42.

Tier One Snack Ideas

Peanut Butter and Celery Sticks

» 2 celery sticks
» 2 T. natural peanut butter

Spoon one tablespoon of peanut butter into each celery stick.

Serves one. Per Serving: calories 188, fat 16, carbs 5, protein 9.

String Cheese Snack

- 2 slices string cheese, low fat

Eat and enjoy!

Serves one. Per Serving: calories 98, fat 4, carbs 1, protein 14.

Nutty Yogurt

- » 1 T. walnut, chopped
- » 6 oz. sugar-free vanilla yogurt

Sprinkle walnuts on top of yogurt and enjoy!

Serves one. Per Serving: calories 98, fat 1, carbs 14, protein 8.

Snackin' Nutz

» 1 oz. almonds or any mixed nuts

Eat and enjoy!

Serves one. Per Serving: calories 167, fat 15, carbs 6, protein 6

Midday Vanilla Smoothies

» 1 c. vanilla soy milk, sugar free
» 1/2 T. vanilla extract
» 1/2 T. Splenda or stevia (sweeten to liking)
» 1/2 c. low-fat cottage cheese
» 1/2 c. egg substitute (Egg Beaters)
» 1/4 tsp. cinnamon, optional

Place all ingredients in a blender and blend until smooth. Add ice cubes (optional).

Serves two. Per Serving: calories 181, fat 10, carbs 6, protein 17.

Chapter Six

Transforming your Body

Welcome to Tier Two

Tier two is designed to broaden your food base. Now that you have gotten through making the shift, we are ready to start adjusting your macronutrient divisions for sustained weight loss at a healthy, consistent, manageable level. During this tier, you are allowed one to two alcoholic beverages per week, but it is not recommended.

In tier two, you will notice some very exciting things taking place. Your cravings will be at a much more manageable level, you'll have better mental focus, and your energy level will be much higher. All of this will be happening simultaneously while many other great, healthy benefits are taking shape, such as the following:

1. Your blood sugar levels will be stabilized.
2. Your water and electrolyte balance will be in check.
3. It will preserve your lean muscle.
4. You will have steady, continued body fat loss.
5. You will maintain a feeling of satiety.

6. It will keep your furnace (metabolism) stoked.
7. It will noticeably improve your blood chemistry.

In the upcoming pages, you will again see a sample day laid out for you as well as recipes labeled in sections: breakfast, lunch, dinner, and snacks. Pick one from each meal category, along with two snacks each day. You will have one serving per meal as well as a snack between meals.

Try to eat approximately every three hours, and *do not* skip meals. Along with your meals, as well as throughout the day, you will need to take in a minimum of two quarts of water. This will continually help flush toxins and fat from your system.

Other allowable beverages are as followed:

Note: A serving equals eight ounces.

- *water, water, water!*
- decaffeinated coffees and teas
- Crystal Light
- sugar-free Kool-Aid
- vegetable juices (no sugar)
- regular coffee and caffeinated diet soda (limit two servings a day)
- skim milk, 1 percent milk, soy milk, and almond milk (limit two servings a day)

Note: If you are stuck in a weight-loss plateau for over two weeks, I encourage you to go back into the tier one process until your weight loss resumes. This does happen to some individuals, which tells me that your metabolism needs a gentle nudge.

Tier Two Sample Day

Let's take a look at a typical day in tier two so you have an understanding of how to structure your meals as well as an idea of the types of foods you will be eating.

Breakfast

Peanut Butter Pancake (page 164)

Snack

Mexi Deviled Eggs (page 254)

Lunch

California Wrap (page 186)

Snack

Tuna Boats (page 257)

Dinner

Grilled Salmon and Cucumber Salad (page 234)

Tier Two Breakfast Recipes

Hash Brown Skillet

» 1 1/5 c. organic hash browns

» 4 oz. organic, low-fat turkey bacon, diced

» 1/2 c. red bell pepper, diced

» 1 c. mushrooms, sliced

» 2 tsp. olive oil

» 4 c. egg whites

» Onion powder

» Salt and pepper

Sauté hash browns, bacon, bell peppers, mushrooms, salt, pepper, and olive oil in nonstick pan over medium-high heat for about seven minutes. Pour in eggs. Season with onion powder, salt, and pepper.

Serves four. Per Serving: calories 321, fat 11, carbs 15.7, protein 36.2.

Greek Yogurt with Almonds

- » 1 6-oz. vanilla nonfat Greek yogurt
- » 10 raw almonds
- » Dash cinnamon
- » Dash nutmeg
- » Dash ground cloves
- » 3 oz. Canadian bacon

Combine yogurt, almonds, and spices. Cook Canadian bacon in a nonstick pan for about two minutes per side.

Serves one. Per Serving: calories 318, fat 12, carbs 16, protein 35.

French Toast with Peanut Butter and Scrambled Eggs

- » 1 slice 100 percent whole wheat bread (15g carbs/slice)
- » 1 1/4 c. egg whites
- » 1 egg
- » 1/2 T. natural peanut butter
- » 1/4 tsp. cinnamon
- » 1/4 tsp. fresh thyme, chopped
- » 1/4 tsp. fresh parsley, chopped
- » Salt and pepper

Pour egg whites into bowl. Soak bread for at least thirty seconds. Cook French toast in a nonstick pan over medium heat, flipping when brown. Remove toast from pan. Sprinkle with cinnamon, and spread with peanut butter. Whip remaining egg whites with whole egg and herbs. Season with salt and pepper. Return to pan and cook, stirring constantly.

Serves one. Per Serving: calories 305, fat 9, carbs 17, protein 39.

Scrambled Breakfast Wrap

- » 1/4 c. red bell pepper, diced
- » 1/4 c. poblano pepper, diced
- » 1/4 c. onion, diced
- » 2 T. olive oil
- » 1/2 c. mushroom, sliced
- » 3 large eggs
- » 1/4 c. celery, diced
- » 1/4 c. tomato, diced

Heat two tablespoons of olive oil in a skillet or electric fry pan and add mushrooms and veggies. Sauté until mushrooms are nicely browned. Beat eggs, a small amount of garlic powder, and black pepper in a bowl. Add eggs to the sautéed veggies, and scramble to your liking. Place in two large lettuce leaves and top with either pesto or salsa (optional). Roll into wrap and enjoy.

Serves one. Per Serving: calories 285, fat 15, carbs 15, protein 22.

Breakfast Flat Bread

» 2 light flat bread
» 4 slices organic low-fat Canadian bacon, diced
» 1 1/2 c. egg whites
» 1/2 c. salsa
» Salt and pepper
» 2 green onions, diced
» 18 almonds

Bake flat bread on oven rack for five to seven minutes at 375 degrees to brown. Season eggs with salt and pepper and cook in nonstick pan over medium heat, stirring the entire time. Remove flat bread from oven. Divide Canadian bacon and eggs among bread. Top with salsa and green onions. Serve with almonds on the side.

Serves one. Per Serving: calories 302, fat 10, carbs 16, protein 37.

Ricotta Pancakes

- » 3 tsp. Splenda or stevia
- » 2 eggs
- » 2 T. low-fat ricotta cheese
- » 1/4 c. nonfat sour cream
- » 1/4 tsp. nutmeg
- » 1/4 tsp. cinnamon
- » 1/4 c. berries of your choice
- » 1 tsp. vanilla extract

Spray skillet with nonstick spray. Mix eggs, ricotta, one teaspoon Splenda or stevia, vanilla, cinnamon, and nutmeg together. Spoon into pan, cook until setting up and then flip, cooking until firm. Mix two teaspoons Splenda or stevia and two tablespoons of water with sour cream and serve over Ricotta pancakes. It can also be topped with sugar-free maple syrup.

Serves one. Per Serving: calories 246, fat 13, carbs 11, protein 20.

Smoked Salmon English muffin

- 2 100 percent whole wheat English muffins
- 24 oz. smoked salmon
- 1/2 English cucumber
- 2 T. Dijon mustard
- 2 T. plain nonfat Greek yogurt
- 1 T. fresh chives, chopped

Divide the salmon among the four English muffin halves. Top with sliced cucumber. Whisk together mustard and Greek yogurt and spoon over cucumber. Top all four with chives.

Serves 4. Per Serving: calories 288, fat 8, carbs 14, protein 35.

Bacon Muffins

- » 1/4 c. red onion, finely chopped
- » 1/4 c. parmesan cheese
- » 1 1/4 c. low-fat mozzarella cheese, thinly sliced
- » 1/2 tsp. Italian seasoning, dried
- » 1 c. egg substitute
- » 4 slices Canadian bacon

Heat oven to 350 degrees. In a large muffin pan, line the bottom of each with Canadian bacon. Mix egg substitute, mozzarella cheese, and Italian seasoning and then pour on top of the Canadian bacon. Sprinkle tops with parmesan cheese and red onion. Bake for fifteen minutes or until set.

Serves four. Per Serving: calories 170, fat 8, carbs 4, protein 18.

Vanilla Smoothie Breakfast

» 1 T. wheat bran
» 1 T. vanilla extract
» 1 c. low-fat yogurt, plain
» 6 ice cubes
» Splenda or stevia to taste

Place all ingredients in a blender and blend until ice is pulverized. Add more ice to thicken as desired.

Serves one. Per Serving: calories 208, fat 4, carbs 25, protein 13.

Oatmeal Cottage Cheese Pancakes

- 1 T. vanilla
- 1/2 c. low-fat cottage cheese
- 1/2 c. rolled oats
- 4 egg whites

Blend all ingredients in a blender. Spray skillet with cooking spray and cook like regular pancakes. Top with sugar-free syrup. Add 1/4 cup of fresh berries of your choice to top it off if you desire.

Serves two. Per Serving: calories 171, fat 2, carbs 18, protein 17.

Oatmeal and Egg Twist

- » 4 egg whites
- » 1 c. water
- » 1/2 c. old-fashioned rolled oats
- » 1 tsp. cinnamon
- » Splenda or stevia to taste

Combine oats, egg whites, water, and cinnamon in a microwave-safe bowl. Microwave for about four minutes in one-minute increments, stirring in between. Let sit for about one minute, then add sweetener and more cinnamon to taste. Top with two tablespoons of crushed walnuts if desired.

Serves one. Per Serving: calories 228, fat 3, carbs 30, protein 21.

Chocolate and Coffee Smoothie

» 1/2 c. oat bran
» 1 c. low-fat yogurt, plain
» 2 T. instant coffee
» 6 ice cubes
» 2 T. cocoa
» Splenda or stevia to taste

Dissolve the instant coffee in two tablespoons of hot water. Dissolve the cocoa in two tablespoons of cold water. When coffee and cocoa are dissolved, blend all ingredients in a blender, sweeten to taste, and serve.

Serves one. Per Serving: calories 312, fat 9, carbs 58, protein 23.

Feta Cheese Omelet

- » 1 1/2 tsp. paprika
- » 2 T. Smart Balance butter
- » 1/2 c. green onion, minced
- » 2 T. fresh dill
- » 4 oz. feta cheese, reduced fat
- » 1 1/2 c. egg substitute
- » Black pepper, freshly ground

If the feta is too salty, soak in cold water for thirty minutes. Drain well, and crumble into fine pieces and combine in a bowl with the scallions and paprika and then set aside. In a large bowl, whisk the egg substitute and pepper together until frothy. Melt the Smart Balance butter in a ten-inch omelet pan over medium heat. When the butter bubbles rapidly, add half of the egg mixture and stir until it just begins to set. Continue cooking until the eggs are almost completely cooked, running a thin spatula around the edges to prevent sticking, for about 1 1/2 minutes. Sprinkle half the feta mixture on the omelet, and then reduce the heat to very low, cover, and cook for one more minute. Slide the omelet onto a plate, folding it over if desired. Repeat with the remaining ingredients, making one more omelet. Serve at once, sprinkled with more paprika and the fresh dill.

Serves two. Per Serving: calories 208, fat 10, carbs 7, protein 21.

Canadian Bacon Egg Cups

- » 2 T. skim milk
- » 2 T. onion, chopped
- » 4 oz. low-fat Monterrey jack cheese, shredded
- » 4 eggs
- » 6 slices Canadian bacon

Cook four slices of the Canadian bacon in a skillet until the center puffs up, about one minute. Put Canadian bacon cups in lightly greased muffin cups. Chop the remaining two slices of bacon. In a small bowl, beat the eggs and milk together. Stir in the chopped Canadian bacon and onion. Pour egg mixture into bacon cups. Bake uncovered in an oven set at 375 degrees for twelve to fifteen minutes or until eggs set. Sprinkle with cheese. Bake for a couple minutes longer, until cheese melts.

Serves four. Per Serving: calories 234, fat 12, carbs 3, protein 26.

Green Tomato-Basil Omelet

- » 3 T. scallion, chopped
- » 1 T. light olive oil, for the pan
- » 6 large eggs
- » 1 lb. green tomato, sliced ½-inch thick
- » 2 T. fresh basil, finely sliced

Fry the tomatoes briefly on each side until they are lightly colored. Don't let them get soft. While the tomatoes are frying, lightly beat the eggs with the scallions and basil. Pour over the tomatoes. Let the eggs sit for about a minute, and then give the pan a shake to loosen the bottom. Cook over medium-low heat until the eggs are nicely colored on the bottom, and then slide the omelet onto a large plate. Place the pan over the plate, invert it, and return to the heat to cook the other side. When done, turn the omelet out onto a serving plate and serve sliced in wedges and garnish with basil.

Serves two. Per Serving: calories 280, fat 15, carbs 14, protein 22.

Mushroom Omelet

» 1/4 c. water
» 2 T. olive oil
» 1/4 lb. mushrooms, cleaned and sliced
» 4 eggs
» 4 egg whites
» 1/2 bell pepper, green or red, chopped

Heat olive oil in a large skillet. Add mushrooms and bell peppers. Cook for five minutes or so, stirring occasionally, until bell pepper is softened. Meanwhile, beat eggs, egg whites, and water in a medium bowl. When vegetables are soft, transfer them to a plate.

Pour the egg mixture into the skillet and cook over medium heat. Lift edges of the skillet to allow raw egg mixture to flow underneath and cook. When the egg is about half set, sprinkle with mushrooms and bell pepper. Fold the egg over to enclose the filling and cook to desired doneness. Slide onto a serving platter, and then divide into portions and serve. Don't be shy about substituting ingredients in the omelet. Season with a little parmesan cheese or other reduced-fat cheeses if desired, or change the vegetable combinations.

Serves two to four. Per Serving: calories 341, fat 25, carbs 7, protein 22.

Quickie Scrambled Eggs and Toast

- » 1 slice multi-grain bread
- » 3 whole eggs

Beat eggs and cook in a nonstick pan to desired consistency. Serve with slice of multi-grain toast, topped with Smart Balance butter or I Can't Believe It's Not Butter. A quick meal for the on the go day!

Serves one. Per Serving: calories 286, fat 16, carbs 13, protein 21.

Quick and Tasty Cottage Cheese

- » 1/2 c. cottage cheese
- » 2 T. chopped almond or walnut
- » Cinnamon to taste
- » Splenda or stevia to taste

Combine cottage cheese, cinnamon, and sweetener and top with walnuts or almonds. Serve with an English muffin topped with peanut butter.

Serves one. Per Serving: calories 318, fat 15, carbs 24, protein 23.

Italian Breakfast Casserole

» 6 slices whole-wheat low-carb bread, cut into 1/2-inch cubes
» 1 c. skim milk
» 1/4 c. reduced-fat cheddar cheese
» 3/4 lb. lean ground pork
» 3/4 tsp. Italian seasoning
» 1/4 tsp. ground red pepper
» 3 green onions, chopped
» 2 garlic cloves, minced
» 1/4 tsp. fennel seed, crushed
» 16 oz. frozen egg substitute, thawed
» 3/4 tsp. dry mustard

Coat a skillet with cooking spray and place over medium-high heat until hot. Add pork, Italian seasoning, fennel seeds, and garlic; cook until meat is browned, stirring to crumble meat. Drain in a colander, pat dry with paper towels, and set aside. Combine milk, cheddar, green onions, dry mustard, and pepper in a large bowl; stir well. Add pork mixture and bread, stirring until just blended. Pour into an eleven-by-seven-by-two-inch baking dish coated with cooking spray. Cover and chill for eight to twelve hours. Bake uncovered at 350 degrees for fifty minutes or until set and lightly browned. Garnish with tomatoes and green onion on top if desired.

Serves six. Per Serving: calories 372, fat 22, carbs 18, protein 23.

Scrambled Breakfast Wrap

» 1/4 c. red bell pepper, diced
» 1/4 c. poblano pepper, diced
» 1/4 c. onion, diced
» 2 T. olive oil
» 1/2 c. mushroom, sliced
» 3 large eggs
» 1/4 c. celery, diced
» 1/4 c. tomato, diced

Heat two tablespoons of olive oil in a skillet or electric fry pan and add mushrooms and veggies. Sauté until mushrooms are nicely browned. Beat eggs, a small amount of garlic powder, and black pepper in a bowl. Add eggs to the sautéed veggies and scramble to your liking. Place in two large lettuce leaves and top with either pesto or salsa (optional). Roll into a wrap and enjoy.

Serves one. Per Serving: calories 285, fat 15, carbs 15, protein 22.

PB Chocolate Cottage Cheese

» 2 tsp. unsweetened cocoa
» 2 T. natural peanut butter
» 1/2 c. low-fat cottage cheese
» 1 tsp. vanilla extract
» Splenda or stevia to taste

Mix all ingredients in a bowl and stir well. Microwave a few seconds to warm up if desired.

Serves one. Per Serving: calories 343, fat 17, carbs 15, protein 23.

Berry Breakfast Smoothie

- » 1 c. vanilla soy milk, sugar free
- » 2 T. Splenda or stevia
- » 6 ice cubes
- » 1/2 c. egg white substitute (Egg Beaters)
- » 1/2 c. berries, frozen (your choice)

Put ingredients in blender and mix until smooth. Add more ice if you wish, to thicken. Enjoy!

Serves one. Per Serving: calories 225, fat 0, carbs 22, protein 32

English Egg, Ham, and Cheese, Please

- 2 whole eggs
- 3 slices Hormel Natural Choice deli ham
- 1 high-fiber English muffin
- 1 oz. low-fat mozzarella cheese

In skillet or electric pan, cook eggs over hard and deli ham until slightly browned. Place eggs and ham topped with cheese on toasted English muffin.

Serves one. Per Serving: calories 335, fat 16, carbs 25, protein 30

Hard-Boiled Egg, English Muffin Breakfast

- » 1/2 grapefruit
- » 1/2 English muffin, mixed grain
- » 1 T. natural peanut butter
- » 3 hardboiled eggs

Toast English muffin and top with peanut butter. Peel hard-boiled eggs. Top grapefruit with either Splenda or stevia sweetener to your liking.

Serves one. Per Serving: calories 453, fat 25, carbs 29, protein 27.

Protein Fruit Bowl

» 1/2 c. vanilla soy milk, sugar free

» 1/2 c. low-fat cottage cheese

» 1/4 c. fresh raspberries or blueberries

» 1/2 c. All-Bran cereal, sugar free

Mix all but berries in a bowl and microwave for 1 1/2 minutes. Serve with berries on top.

Serves one. Per Serving: calories 222, fat 5, carbs 33, protein 21

Olive Salmon Scramble

» 1/4 c. skim milk
» 2 oz. shallots, finely chopped
» 1 lb. salmon fillet, cut into chunks
» 2 oz. reduced-fat mozzarella cheese
» 2 T. olive oil
» 2 T. Dijon mustard
» 1/4 tsp. black pepper
» 1 c. black olives, drained
» 2 oz. arugula, stems removed
» 8 eggs

In a large mixing bowl, whisk together eggs, milk, mustard, and pepper and then set aside. Heat one tablespoon of olive oil in a large nonstick pan over medium-high heat. Add salmon and cook for three to five minutes, turning occasionally until browned and cooked through. Place cooked salmon on a plate and set aside. Heat remaining oil in a clean pan over high heat. Add shallots and cook for 1 minute. Pour eggs in and cook for three to five minutes, stirring occasionally until set. Turn heat to medium-low and fold in olives, cheese, arugula, and salmon.

Serves six. Per Serving: calories 294, fat 18, carbs 5, protein 28.

All-Bran Pancake

- » 3 eggs
- » 1/4 tsp. cinnamon
- » 1/2 c. All-Bran cereal

Place all ingredients in a blender and blend. Heat skillet sprayed with cooking spray over medium-high heat. Pour batter into skillet, and flip when edges are golden. Serve with sugar-free maple syrup.

Serves one. Per Serving: calories 306, fat 16, carbs 25, protein 23.

Peanut Butter Pancake

- » 2 tsp. skim milk
- » 1/2 c. rolled oats
- » 1 T. natural peanut butter
- » 1/4 c. low-fat cottage cheese
- » 1 egg
- » 1/4 tsp. vanilla extract

Put rolled oats in a blender and process on high for one minute. In a medium bowl, mix all ingredients together. Cook on a skillet over medium-high heat coated in cooking spray. Cook until both sides are golden. Serve with sugar-free maple syrup or sugar-free fruit preserves.

Serves one. Per Serving: calories 382, fat 16, carbs 33, protein 24.

Chocolate Flax Porridge

- » 1 tsp. vanilla extract
- » 1 T. unsweetened cocoa
- » 1 T. Splenda or stevia
- » 1/4 c. fresh raspberries or strawberries
- » 1/2 c. flaxseed, ground
- » 1/2 tsp. cinnamon
- » 1/4 c. walnut, toasted
- » 2 c. water

Combine all ingredients, except fruit and nuts, in a saucepan. Simmer on low heat until hot and bubbling, stirring frequently. Add more water until it's the consistency you desire. Spoon into bowl and top with nuts and fruit.

Serves two. Per Serving: calories 308, fat 22, carbs 19, protein 12

Mushroom Omelet

» 1/4 c. water

» 2 T. olive oil

» 1/4 lb. mushrooms, cleaned and sliced

» 4 egg whites

» 4 eggs

» 1/2 bell pepper, green or red, chopped

Heat olive oil in a large skillet, and sauté mushrooms and bell pepper. Cook for five minutes, until soft, and transfer to a plate. Pour eggs into skillet and cook until almost set, and then add vegetables and fold egg over to enclose veggies. Cook until desired doneness and sprinkle with cheese (optional).

Serves four. Per Serving: calories 287, fat 21, carbs 9, protein 16

Spinach, Mushroom, and Rice Frittata

- 1 c. wild rice
- 3 1/2 c. egg whites
- 6 eggs
- 2 oz. reduced-fat feta cheese
- 1/2 c. frozen spinach, squeezed
- 1/4 c. red onion, chopped
- 1/2 c. mushrooms, sliced
- 2 tsp. fresh thyme
- Hot sauce
- Salt and pepper

Cook rice. Set one cup aside to cool. Whisk together egg whites and eggs. Combine all ingredients using hot sauce, salt, and pepper to taste. Pour into an oven-safe dish. Bake at 375 degrees for thirty to forty-five minutes or until eggs are set.

Serves four. Per Serving: calories 291, fat 9.5, carbs 13, protein 35.7

Peanut Butter Protein Shake

» 24 oz. vanilla nonfat Greek yogurt
» 4 T. natural peanut butter
» 3 scoops 100 percent whey protein powder
» Water

Combine all ingredients in blender. Add water if desired.

Serves four. Per Serving: calories 322, fat 10, carbs 17, protein 38.

Peanut Butter Pancake with Canadian Bacon

- » 1/4 c. plain organic oatmeal
- » 1/4 c. 1 percent fat cottage cheese
- » 1/2 c. egg whites
- » 1/2 T. natural peanut butter
- » 3 slices Canadian bacon

Combine the first four ingredients in a blender. Blend until smooth. Heat a small, nonstick pan over medium heat. Pour mixture into pan. Cover with lid. When top of pancake is set completely, flip. Cook the second side for one minute. Remove from pan. Cook Canadian bacon until warm. Serve together.

Serves one. Per Serving: calories 327, fat 12, carbs 17, protein 34.4.

Vegan Tofu Scrambler

- » 1/2 tsp. turmeric
- » 1/2 green bell pepper, chopped
- » 1 pack low-fat Mori-Nu brand firm tofu, crumbled
- » 1/2 medium onion, chopped
- » 1 T. minced garlic
- » 1 T. olive oil
- » 1/8 tsp. cumin
- » 2 T. Braggs liquid amino

Preheat olive oil in a large saucepan over medium-high heat. Add onions and garlic and sauté until translucent. Add tofu, turmeric, cumin, and Braggs; mix together. Sauté on medium-high heat for five to ten minutes until moisture has evaporated. Add some Gimme Lean sausage style soy if desired.

Serves one. Per Serving: calories 255, fat 19, carbs 12, protein 11.

Strawberry Tofu Smoothie

» 1 c. sugar-free soy milk or skim milk

» 1 c. frozen strawberry

» 1/4 c. tofu

» Splenda or stevia to taste

Throw all ingredients into a blender and mix. Enjoy!

Serves one. Per Serving: calories 187, fat 4, carbs 27, protein 14.

Broccoli Cheese Casserole

» 1/4 c. skim milk

» 8 oz. low-fat turkey sausage

» 1 c. low-fat ricotta cheese

» 1 1/2 c. low-fat cheddar cheese

» 10 oz. frozen broccoli florets, chopped

» 2 c. egg substitute

» 1 tsp. black pepper

» 2 roma tomatoes, thinly sliced

Place sausage in a large, deep skillet. Cook over medium-high heat until evenly browned. Drain, crumble, and set aside. Preheat oven to 350 degrees. Spray a seven-by-eleven-inch baking dish with cooking spray. In a bowl mix sausage, broccoli (thawed and drained), and 1/2 cup cheddar cheese. In a separate bowl, mix 1/2 cup cheddar cheese, ricotta, egg, milk, and pepper. Spoon sausage mixture into prepared baking dish. Spread the ricotta mixture over sausage mixture. Sprinkle remaining cheddar cheese on, and arrange tomato slices on top. Cover with aluminum foil and bake thirty minutes. Uncover and bake an additional fifteen minutes. Let stand ten minutes before serving.

Serves six. Per Serving: calories 237, fat 13, carbs 6, protein 24.

Tier Two
Lunch Recipes

Chicken Fajitas

- » 20 oz. chicken breast cut in strips
- » 1/2 onion, cut in rings
- » 1 red pepper cut in strips
- » 1 1/2 T. olive oil
- » 2 tsp. ground cumin
- » 1 tsp. ground oregano
- » 2 tsp. garlic powder
- » 2 tsp. onion powder
- » 2 tsp. chili powder
- » 1 tsp. red pepper flakes
- » 1 tsp. black pepper
- » 1 tsp. salt
- » 4 low-carb tortillas

Sauté chicken breast, onion, bell pepper, and olive oil in nonstick pan, over medium-high heat until chicken is cooked through. Add dry seasonings, and stir together completely. Remove from heat and serve in tortillas.

Serves four. Per Serving: calories 321, fat 10, carbs 15, protein 38.

Chicken Salad with Grapes and Walnuts

- 4 oz. chicken breast, shredded
- 1 1/2 T. plain nonfat Greek yogurt
- 1 1/2 T. Dijon mustard
- 15 grapes, halved
- 7 walnut halves, chopped
- 2 tsp. tarragon
- 2 tsp. fresh lemon juice
- Salt and pepper
- Hot sauce

Combine all ingredients, seasoning with salt, pepper, and hot sauce to taste.

Serves one. Per Serving: calories 310, fat 12, carbs 12, protein 34.

Thai Chicken-Stuffed Mushrooms

» 18 oz. chicken breast, diced
» 1 clove garlic, chopped
» 3/4 c. rice noodles
» 4 portabella mushrooms
» 1/4 c. natural peanut butter
» 3 T. low-sodium soy sauce
» 1/2 lemon, juiced
» 2 tsp. ground ginger
» Salt and pepper
» 3 green onions, chopped

Cook chicken breast and garlic in nonstick pan over medium heat until juices run clear. Cook rice noodles as directed. Set aside 3/4 cup. Bake portabella mushrooms, seasoned with salt and pepper, in oven at 375 degrees for ten to fifteen minutes. Remove from pan and set aside. When chicken is cooked, add noodles to pan as well as peanut butter, soy, lemon juice, ginger, salt, and pepper. Toss to coat and heat through. Divide mixture among mushrooms and top with green onions.

Serves four. Per Serving: calories 323, fat 11, carbs 16.6, protein 36.3.

BBQ Pork

» 16 oz. pork tenderloin

» Pickle juice

» 1/2 c. BBQ sauce

» 1/2 c. ketchup

» 2 T. garlic chili sauce

» 4 c. broccoli

» 1 1/2 T. olive oil

» Seasoned black pepper

» Salt and pepper

Cook pork tenderloin in slow cooker with pickle juice (add water if tenderloin is not covered) for five to seven hours. Combine BBQ sauce, ketchup, and garlic chili paste in bowl. Sauté broccoli and olive oil, in nonstick pan, over medium-high heat for about seven minutes. Season with seasoned black pepper. Serve tenderloin with a side of BBQ sauce and broccoli.

Serves four. Per Serving: calories 318, fat 11, carbs 16, protein 35.

Salsa Turkey Burgers

- 1/2 c. salsa (mild or spicy)
- 5 whole wheat low-carb buns
- 2 Italian turkey sausages, casing removed
- 1 lb. ground turkey breast
- 1/3 c. flaxseed, ground
- 1 egg

Mix all together in a large bowl and form into patties. Can either grill or pan fry in nonstick pan. Optional: sliced tomato, sliced onion, sugar-free ketchup (Hunts makes an excellent-tasting sugar-free ketchup), low-fat cheese, sliced jalapenos, or veggie topping of your choice. Try a side salad or steamed veggies to accompany if desired.

Serves five. Per Serving: calories 339, fat 16, carbs 20, protein 28

Quickie Lunch Pizza

» 1/4 c. soy pepperoni slices

» 1/4 c. pizza sauce, sugar free

» 1/4 c. low-fat mozzarella cheese, shredded

» 1 low-carb whole wheat tortilla

Heat a large skillet with cooking spray over medium-high heat. Place tortilla on the skillet and spoon sauce evenly over half of tortilla. Next place the pepperoni slices evenly and then the cheese. Fold tortilla over, and heat each side until golden. A nice, quick, light pizza lunch on the go!

Serves one. Per Serving: calories 280, fat 12, carbs 24, protein 20.

Chicken Wrap

» 6 low-carb whole wheat tortillas
» 1/3 c. light mayonnaise
» 6 c. lettuce, shredded
» 2 jalapeno chili peppers, chopped
» 6 hardboiled eggs, chopped
» 3 T. Dijon mustard
» 4 1/2 c. chicken breast, cooked and shredded
» 1/2 c. pecans, chopped
» 1/3 c. red onion, finely chopped
» 1/3 c. roma tomato, chopped

Mix together mayo, mustard, tomato, onion, eggs (optional), and jalapeno. Add chicken. Divide mixture evenly and spread on six tortillas. Sprinkle with lettuce and pecans, and roll up.

Serves six. Per Serving: calories 405, fat 18, carbs 32, protein 30.

Bulgur and Beef

- » 1 c. tomato, chopped
- » 2 c. low-sodium beef broth
- » 1 lb. lean ground beef
- » 2 green onions, chopped
- » 1 T. garlic, minced
- » 2 sticks celery, diced
- » 1 tsp. cayenne pepper
- » 1 c. bulgur wheat, uncooked

Place ground beef in a nonstick skillet over medium-high heat. Crumble beef and cook until almost done. Drain any grease, and stir in celery, onions, tomato, garlic, and cayenne. Cook until celery is tender. Bring beef broth to a boil in a separate pan. Add the bulgur wheat, cover, and reduce to low. Simmer ten minutes or until tender. Stir into beef mixture, and enjoy a comforting meal!

Serves four. Per Serving: calories 405, fat 17, carbs 32, protein 33.

Tuna Melt Muffin

- » 6 oz. tuna in water, drained
- » 1oz. reduced-fat cheddar cheese
- » 1 T. light mayonnaise
- » 1/8 tsp. garlic powder
- » 1/2 tsp. dried minced onion
- » 1 whole wheat English muffin

Mix tuna, mayo, onion, and garlic. Divide tuna mixture on top of each muffin half, and sprinkle with cheese. Toast muffin in toaster oven or regular oven (preheated to 350 degrees) for five to seven minutes until cheese is melted and toasty!

Serves two. Per Serving: calories 216, fat 5, carbs 16, protein 26.

Open-Faced Tuna Steak Sandwiches

- » 4 4-oz. yellow fin tuna fillets
- » 1/4 c. egg whites
- » 1/4 c. panko bread crumbs
- » 2 1/2 T. olive oil
- » 2 T. wasabi mustard
- » 1 T. low-sodium soy sauce
- » 1 T. pickle relish
- » 2 c. spinach
- » 2 100 percent whole wheat sandwich thins

Pour egg whites in bowl. Pour bread crumbs in separate bowl. Dip tuna fillets in egg white and then into crumbs. Set aside coated fillets. Heat olive oil in nonstick skillet over medium-high heat. Place fillets in oil and sear for two minutes on each side. Remove from pan. Whisk together mustard, soy sauce, and relish. Top sandwich thin halves with spinach, place tuna fillet on lettuce, and top with relish.

Serves four. Per Serving: calories 303, fat 10, carbs 13, protein 38.

Buffalo Chicken Pasta

» 16 oz. chicken breast, cut in chunks

» 1/2 c. Louisiana hot sauce

» 1 clove garlic, diced

» 1 1/2 T. olive oil

» 1 1/4 c. cooked, organic pasta

» 4 oz. reduced-fat feta cheese

» 1/3 c. plain nonfat Greek yogurt

» 3 green onions, diced

» 2 T. chives, diced

» 1/2 lemon, juiced

» Salt and pepper

Sauté chicken breast, hot sauce, garlic, and olive oil in nonstick pan, over medium heat, until juices run clear. Cook pasta and set aside 1 1/4 cups. Combine all ingredients.

Serves four. Per Serving: calories 318, fat 11, carbs 16, protein 35.

Grilled Chicken Sandwich

» 5 oz. chicken breast

» Garlic powder, onion powder, salt, and pepper

» 1 T. balsamic vinegar

» 1/5 tsp. olive oil

» 1/2 100 percent whole wheat sandwich thin

» 1/2 oz. pancetta

» 1 tomato slice

Season chicken breast with seasonings to taste. Sauté chicken breast, balsamic vinegar, and olive oil in nonstick pan, over medium heat, until juices run clear. Remove from pan and place on sandwich thin. Cook pancetta for a few minutes and place on top of chicken. Top with sliced tomato.

Serves four. Per Serving: calories 302, fat 10, carbs 13, protein 38.

California Wrap

- 1/4 c. alfalfa sprout
- 1/2 avocado
- 1 1/2 low-carb whole wheat tortilla
- 2 tomatoes, sliced
- 1 T. salsa
- 2 oz. turkey, thinly sliced

Mash avocado and add salsa. Spread avocado mixture over tortilla, leaving an inch around the outside. Add turkey, alfalfa sprouts, and sliced tomatoes. Carefully roll the tortilla into a wrap and slice in half if desired.

Serves one. Per Serving: calories 379, fat 19, carbs 37, protein 20.

Tuna Wrap

- » 1/4 c. lettuce, shredded
- » 1 low-carb whole wheat tortilla
- » 2 tsp. Dijon mustard
- » 1 T. low-fat mayonnaise
- » 1 tsp. lemon juice
- » 1 T. caper
- » 3 oz. albacore tuna in water, drained

Combine tuna, mayonnaise, mustard, and lemon juice. Spread tuna mixture over wrap, and add lettuce with capers. Roll up and enjoy!

Serves one. Per Serving: calories 286, fat 7, carbs 30, protein 26.

Curry Crab Salad

» 2 low-carb whole wheat tortillas
» 1/3 c. light mayonnaise
» 1/4 tsp. curry powder
» 8 oz. crab meat
» 1/4 c. celery, finely chopped
» 1/4 tsp. black pepper
» 1 T. mustard
» 1 onion, finely chopped

In a bowl, mix all ingredients and let sit in fridge for one hour to let flavors blend. Divide into tortillas (optional) and roll up, or serve over greens. Enjoy!

Serves two. Per Serving: calories 375, fat 12, carbs 38, protein 29

Simple Shrimp Salad

- » 1 lb. shrimp, cooked, peeled, and deveined
- » 3 hardboiled eggs, chopped
- » 1/2 c. light mayonnaise
- » 1/2 onion, finely chopped
- » 1/8 tsp. celery salt
- » 1/8 tsp. creole seasoning

Place shrimp in a food processor and pulse until finely minced. Transfer to a bowl, and add eggs, along with other ingredients. Mix well and chill. Divide and serve on greens or a whole wheat tortilla wrap.

Serves four. Per Serving: calories 245, fat 11, carbs 6, protein 29

California Pita Pocket

» 1/4 c. light mayonnaise

» 2 c. lettuce, shredded

» 1 c. picante sauce, no sugar added

» 2 avocados, peeled, pitted, and diced

» 2 c. chicken breast, cooked and finely chopped

» 1/4 c. red onion, diced

» 1/4 c. black olive, sliced

» 3/4 c. reduced fat Monterrey jack cheese

» 1 tomato, diced

» 3 whole wheat pita, halved

Combine half of the picante sauce and the mayo; mix well. Toss with lettuce, avocado, tomato, chicken, olives, and onion. Spoon into pita pockets, top with grated cheese, and drizzle with remaining picante sauce. To warm pita bread, wrap in foil and bake at 250 degrees for ten minutes.

Serves six. Per Serving: calories 387, fat 20, carbs 26, protein 28.

Tuna Quesadilla

» 1/2 c. spinach leaf, fresh
» 1/4 c. salsa, no sugar added
» 1 T. low-fat mayonnaise
» 1/2 c. low-fat cheddar cheese
» 4 low-carb whole wheat tortillas
» 1 tsp. cumin
» 6 oz. canned tuna, water packed, drained

Chop fresh spinach. In a bowl combine tuna, salsa, mayo, cumin, cheese, and spinach. Heat a large skillet over medium-high heat with cooking spray. Lay one whole tortilla down on heated skillet, and spread half of the tuna mixture evenly over tortilla. Place second tortilla on top. Cook two to three minutes or until browned and flip, browning other side. Repeat with last two tortillas and tuna mixture. Slice quesadillas and serve with optional low-fat sour cream and additional salsa if desired.

Serves two. Per Serving: calories 328, fat 5, carbs 26, protein 37.

Shrimp with White Beans

» 16 oz. raw shrimp
» 8 oz. organic, low-fat chicken sausage
» 2 tsp. olive oil
» 2 oz. orange juice
» 1 red bell pepper, diced
» 1/4 c. onion, diced
» 1 clove garlic, minced
» 1/2 c. mushrooms, diced
» Salt and pepper
» 1 c. great northern beans, drained and rinsed
» 1 T. fresh basil, chopped

Sauté shrimp, chicken sausage, olive oil, orange juice, pepper, onion, garlic, mushrooms, salt, and pepper in nonstick pan over medium-high heat for about seven minutes or until shrimp are no longer translucent. Add beans, and stir in gently. Garnish with fresh basil.

Serves four. Per Serving: calories 286, fat 9, carbs 14, protein 35

Strawberry and Walnut Pita

- » 1 T. walnut, chopped
- » 1/4 c. strawberry
- » 3/4 c. low-fat cottage cheese
- » 1 whole wheat pita, halved

Mix together cottage cheese, strawberries (sliced), and walnuts. Place in 1/2 toasted pita pocket and enjoy!

Serves one. Per Serving: calories 251, fat 7, carbs 23, protein 26.

Beef and Spinach Pita Pocket

» 8 oz. lean ground beef

» 2 tsp. garlic

» 1/4 tsp. crushed red pepper

» 1 1/2 c. spinach, fresh and torn

» 1/4 tsp. cumin

» 1/4 tsp. coriander

» 1/8 tsp. ginger

» 6 spinach leaves, fresh

» 1 whole wheat pita, halved

» 2 T. low-fat plain yogurt

» 1/8 tsp. curry powder

In a large, nonstick skillet, combine ground beef, garlic, and crushed red pepper. Cook over medium heat until browned, stirring to crumble beef. Drain. Add chopped spinach and spices, and stir well. Cover and cook over medium heat for three minutes or until spinach is wilted. Remove from heat. Spoon half of the beef mixture into each pita half lined with whole spinach leaves. Mix yogurt with (optional) curry powder. Top each half with one tablespoon of yogurt mixture or plain yogurt.

Serves two. Per Serving: calories 361, fat 20, carbs 19, protein 27.

Avocado Tuna Wrap

- 1 low-carb whole wheat tortilla
- 1 tsp. lemon juice
- 1 T. flaxseed, ground
- ½ cucumber, peeled, seeded, and chopped
- 1/2 avocado
- 2 oz. tuna in water, drained

Mash avocado. Mix all ingredients together and place in center of tortilla. Roll up and enjoy!

Serves one. Per Serving: calories 451, fat 24, carbs 41, protein 22.

Oriental Lettuce Wraps

» 1 tsp. sambal oelek (or more)
» 1 T. reduced-sodium soy sauce
» 1/2 c. red bell pepper, chopped
» Parmesan cheese (optional)
» 1 T. oyster sauce
» 1 onion, chopped
» 1 lb. lean ground beef
» 1 T. garlic
» 1/4 c. cucumber, peeled, seeded, and chopped
» 4 crisp lettuce leaves

Spray skillet with nonstick spray and add ground beef, onion, and garlic. Cook until beef is almost cooked through, about five to six minutes. Add cucumber and red pepper and cook for five minutes. Add soy sauce, oyster sauce, and sambal oelek. Mix well and reduce mixture to about half. Place four tablespoons of mixture on a lettuce leaf, roll, and serve. Sprinkle with parmesan cheese if desired.

Serves four. Per Serving: calories 290, fat 19, carbs 5, protein 22.

Chicken and Walnut Salad

» 1/4 c. walnut, chopped
» 1 bag mixed salad greens
» 3 T. extra-virgin olive oil
» 1 tsp. dried basil
» 2 cooked chicken breasts
» 3 T. balsamic vinegar

In a saucepan, combine olive oil, balsamic vinegar, basil, and walnuts. Cook until somewhat thickened and liquid is reduced. Place greens on salad dish, and place chicken on top. Drizzle with dressing.

Serves two. Per Serving: calories 410, fat 31, carbs 4, protein 31.

Citrus Soy Bean Salad

- » 1/4 c. scallions, chopped
- » 1/4 tsp. salt
- » 3/4 c. reduced-fat Monterrey jack cheese
- » 1 T. olive oil
- » 1/4 c. lime juice
- » 2 tsp. jalapeno pepper, minced
- » 1/2 tsp. cumin
- » 3 T. cilantro, chopped
- » 1 c. bulgur wheat
- » 1 15-oz. can black soybeans, drained
- » 1 c. water, boiling
- » 1 1/2 c. zucchini, diced

Combine bulgur and boiling water in a large bowl and stir well. Cover and let stand for thirty minutes or until liquid is absorbed. Add zucchini and soy beans, stirring gently. Then add cheeses, cilantro, and scallions. In a separate bowl, combine orange juice and remaining ingredients and stir well. Pour dressing over bulgur mixture and toss gently. Serve at room temperature or chilled.

Serves four. Per Serving: calories 416, fat 16, carbs 6, protein 28

Lemon Basil Chicken Salad

- » 2 T. lemon juice
- » 1 lb. chicken breast, cooked and finely chopped
- » 2 celery sticks rib, finely chopped
- » 2 T. basil, fresh and chopped
- » 1/4 c. low-fat mayonnaise
- » 1/2 tsp. salt
- » 1/2 c. sour cream, light

Combine sour cream, mayonnaise, basil, lemon juice, salt, and pepper. Add chicken and celery. Serve over salad greens or in a whole wheat low-carb wrap.

Serves four. Per Serving: calories 249, fat 12, carbs 4, protein 30.

Canadian Bacon Spinach Salad

- » 8 c. spinach, fresh and torn
- » 1/2 c. peanut s
- » 2 tsp. orange zest
- » 1/2 c. orange juice
- » 2 hardboiled eggs, chopped
- » 1 golden delicious apple, diced
- » 1 c. celery, thinly sliced
- » 6 oz. Canadian bacon, sliced into narrow strips
- » 1 tsp. Splenda or stevia
- » 1 c. sugar-free vanilla yogurt

In a small bowl, mix dressing ingredients: yogurt, sweetener, orange zest, and orange juice. In a large bowl, mix salad ingredients—spinach, Canadian bacon, eggs, celery, apple, and peanuts—and then toss. Combine dressing with salad and toss well. Enjoy!

Serves four. Per Serving: calories 273, fat 15, carbs 16, protein 21

Tasty Meatball Wrap

- » 8 oz. reduced-fat Monterrey jack cheese
- » 1/4 c. parmesan cheese, grated
- » 1/4 c. old-fashioned rolled oats
- » 6 low-carb whole wheat tortillas
- » 2 Italian turkey sausages, casing removed
- » 1 lb. ground turkey breast
- » 1 egg
- » 2 T. basil pesto
- » 1 jar spaghetti sauce, no sugar added

Combine in a bowl turkey breast, turkey sausage, pesto, parmesan, egg, and oatmeal. Form into meatballs (around eighteen). Heat a deep nonstick skillet over medium-high heat with cooking spray. Add meatballs, and brown on all sides. Then add spaghetti sauce, and lower heat. Simmer or twenty minutes. Place three meatballs with some sauce down the center of each tortilla and top with one to two ounces of shredded cheese. Roll up and enjoy.

Serves six. Per Serving: calories 496, fat 22, carbs 32, protein 34

Strawberry Cottage Cheese

» 1/2 c. low-fat cottage cheese
» 1 T. flaxseed, ground
» 1/2 c. Fiber One cereal
» 1/2 c. strawberry
» Splenda or stevia to taste

Slice strawberries and mix with the rest of the ingredients. Enjoy!

Serves one. Per Serving: calories 212, fat 6, carbs 36, protein 18

Jicama Chicken Salad

- » 4 cooked chicken breasts
- » 1/2 jicama, peeled and sliced into matchstick slices
- » 3 navel oranges, peeled and sliced thin
- » 1 bag romaine lettuce greens
- » 1/4 c. toasted pecans, chopped
- » 1/4 c. olive oil
- » 2 T. red wine vinegar
- » 1 tsp. honey
- » 1 tsp. garlic, minced

In a bowl, mix chopped pecans, olive oil, red wine vinegar, honey, and garlic. In a second bowl, toss jicama, oranges, and greens. Portion greens onto plates and top each with a sliced chicken breast. Top with dressing mixture from first bowl.

Serves four. Per Serving: calories 381, fat 20, carbs 22, protein 30.

Salmon Muffins

- 1/2 c. rolled oats
- 2 tsp. lemon juice
- 1/4 c. evaporated milk, low fat
- 1/2 c. celery, chopped
- 1/4 tsp. black pepper
- 1/2 tsp. baking powder
- 1 6-oz. can salmon, not drained
- Tabasco sauce, to taste

Preheat oven to 350 degrees. Add all ingredients; puree until well blended. Spoon batter into preheated muffin tins, dividing evenly. Bake for thirty minutes or until golden. (Optional—sprinkle with low-fat cheese last five minutes of baking.)

Serves two. Per Serving: calories 265, fat 8, carbs 18, protein 29.

Hero-Style Wrap

» 2 slices low-fat Swiss cheese
» 2 low-carb whole wheat tortillas
» 1 T. light mayonnaise
» 2 lettuce leaves
» 4 slices fat-free turkey
» 4 slices fat-free ham, deli-style
» 1 T. Dijon mustard
» 1 c. alfalfa sprouts
» 1 tomato, sliced

Mix together mayo and Dijon mustard. Place a tablespoon of mixture on each tortilla. Divide and place lettuce leaves, turkey, ham, and cheese on each tortilla. Top with tomatoes and alfalfa sprouts and roll up. Serve or wrap in plastic and refrigerate until ready to eat.

Serves two. Per Serving: calories 387, fat 12, carbs 34, protein 34

Tuna Muffins

- » 2 oz. reduced-fat cheddar cheese
- » 2 T. onion, finely chopped
- » 1tsp Old Bay seasoning
- » 1/4 c. green bell pepper, minced
- » 2 eggs
- » 1/4 c. celery, finely chopped
- » 2 6-oz. cans tuna, water packed and drained

Preheat oven to 350 degrees. Mix ingredients together and spoon into six well-greased muffin cups. Bake for thirty minutes or until browned around the edges.

Serves three. Per Serving: calories 209, fat 6, carbs 2, protein 35.

Vegetarian Chickpea Salad

» 1 T. parmesan cheese, grated
» 1 T. olive oil
» 1 c. grape tomato, halved
» 1 T. garlic, minced
» 1 15.5-oz can garbanzo beans, drained and rinsed
» 1/2 tsp. dried parsley
» 1/2 tsp. dried basil
» 1 cucumber, peeled, seeded, and chopped
» 3 T. balsamic vinegar
» 1/4 c. red onion, finely chopped
» 1/4 tsp. salt

For the dressing, combine olive oil, balsamic vinegar, and salt in a small bowl. Combine all other ingredients in a bowl, pour the dressing over, and toss gently. Cover and refrigerate for at least one hour. Serve chilled and over salad greens.

Serves four. Per Serving: calories 245, fat 7, carbs 37, protein 11

Asian-Style Chicken Slaw

- » 2 T. Splenda or stevia
- » 1/4 c. slivered almonds, toasted
- » 1/4 c. rice wine vinegar
- » 1 T. reduced-sodium soy sauce
- » 1/2 c. red bell pepper, finely chopped
- » 10-oz. package shredded cabbage
- » 1/4 c. onion, finely chopped
- » 1/4 c. cider vinegar
- » 1 lb. chicken breast, cooked and shredded
- » 3/4 c. celery, finely chopped
- » 1/4 tsp. black pepper
- » 1/2 c. sugar snap pea, chopped
- » 1 tsp. toasted sesame seeds
- » 1 8-oz. can water chestnuts, drained

To prepare slaw, combine the chicken, celery, peas, bell peppers, onions, cabbage, and water chestnuts ingredients in a bowl. Combine dressing ingredients—cider vinegar, rice wine vinegar, sweetener, soy sauce, and pepper—in separate bowl. Pour dressing over slaw mixture, and toss to coat. Garnish with slivered almonds and toasted sesame seeds. Cover and chill for at least one hour. Sprinkle with toasted almonds and sesame seeds.

Serves four. Per Serving: calories 236, fat 7, carbs 10, protein 31.

Cilantro Crab Salad

- » 1 c. sour cream, light
- » 1/2 red bell pepper, chopped
- » 1 lime, juiced
- » 1/2 c. green chili, diced
- » 1/4 c. garlic powder
- » 1/4 tsp. cumin
- » 1 lb. crab meat
- » 1/4 c. cilantro, chopped

Combine sour cream, red bell pepper, chilies, cilantro, lime juice, and garlic powder in a bowl. Add crab meat and chill for at least one hour. Serve over salad greens. Garnish with carrot curls (optional).

Serves four. Per Serving: calories 147, fat 3, carbs 5, protein 25.

Tier Two
Dinner Recipes

Asian Meatloaf

- 16 oz. extra-lean ground turkey
- 1 organic egg, beaten
- 4 oz. reduced-fat feta cheese
- 4 green onions, chopped
- 1 clove garlic, chopped
- 2 T. garlic chili paste
- 1/2 c. soy sauce
- 1 1/2 c. wild rice, cooked
- 1 1/2 T. olive oil
- Salt and pepper

Cook rice and set aside 1 1/2 cups. Combine all ingredients in a large bowl. Wearing disposable gloves, mix meatloaf with hands. Place in a baking dish or baking pan and shape as desired. Bake uncovered for thirty-five to forty-five minutes or until cooked through.

Serves four. Per Serving: calories 311, fat 11, carbs 15, protein 37.

Cod with Prosciutto and Chickpeas

» 20 oz. cod
» 1 c. chickpeas, drained and rinsed
» 1 T. olive oil
» 1 lemon, juiced
» 1 c. mushrooms, diced
» 1 clove garlic, pressed
» 3 T. capers
» 2 ½ oz. prosciutto, diced
» 2 tsp. fresh thyme
» Old Bay seasoning
» Salt and pepper

Place fish fillets in glass baking dish. Disperse chickpeas around fish. Drizzle fish with olive oil. Scatter lemon juice, mushrooms, garlic, capers, prosciutto, and thyme over fish and beans. Season to taste with Old Bay, salt, and pepper.

Serves four. Per Serving: calories 304, fat 8, carbs 18, protein 39.

Lobster and Shrimp Salad

- » 12 oz. lobster tails
- » 9 oz. raw shrimp
- » 2 cloves garlic, diced
- » 1/2 jalapeño pepper, diced
- » 2 limes, juiced
- » 2 T. red pepper flakes
- » 2 T. olive oil
- » Salt and pepper
- » 1 c. corn
- » 1/4 c. mayo with olive oil
- » 1/4 c. plain nonfat Greek yogurt
- » 3 green onions, diced
- » 2 T. fresh cilantro, chopped

Cut lobster tails out of shell and cut into chunks. Cut raw shrimp into similar-size chunks. Sauté lobster, shrimp, garlic, jalapeño, lime juice, red pepper flakes, olive oil, salt, and pepper in nonstick pan over medium-high heat for about seven minutes or until lobster and shrimp are no longer translucent. Remove from heat. In bowl, stir together seafood mixture, corn, mayo, Greek yogurt, and green onions. Season, again, with salt and pepper to taste. Garnish with cilantro.

Serves four. Per Serving: calories 322, fat 13, carbs 15, protein 36.

Chicken and Carrots Grill Packs

- 20 oz. chicken breast
- 1 lemon, juiced
- 1 1/2 c. organic carrots, sliced
- 1 1/2 c. organic celery, chopped
- 1/2 c. onion, sliced
- 2 T. olive oil
- Garlic powder
- salt and pepper
- 1 oz. asiago cheese
- 2 T. fresh parsley, chopped

Tear off generous aluminum foil squares for chicken breasts. Place chicken in center of foil. Fold up corners slightly to create an area to work with. Divide lemon juice, carrots, celery, and onion among chicken. Drizzle with oil. Season with garlic powder, salt, and pepper. Grill for fifteen to twenty minutes. Remove from foils, and top with cheese and parsley.

Serves: Per Serving: calories 298, fat 12, carbs 11, protein 36

Vegetarian Greek Spaghetti Squash

» 2 c. tomato, chopped

» 3 c. spaghetti squash, cooked and shredded

» 1/2 c. reduced-fat feta cheese

» 3 T. red wine vinegar

» 1/4 c. red onion, thinly sliced

» 1 tsp. oregano, dried

» 1/4 red bell pepper, diced

» 1 T. garlic, minced

» 1 15-oz. can garbanzo bean, drained

» 1 T. extra-virgin olive oil

» 1 c. cucumber, peeled, seeded, and diced

» 1/4 c. black olive, sliced

» 1 tsp. basil, dried

» 1 tsp. balsamic vinegar

» 1/4 tsp. black pepper

In a bowl, combine vinegars, oil, oregano, basil, black pepper, and garlic. Whisk well. In another bowl, combine cooked squash, tomato, cucumber, feta cheese, bell pepper, onion, olives, and garbanzo beans. Add whisked dressing and toss well. Cover and chill at least one hour.

Serves four. Per Serving: calories 321, fat 10, carbs 48, protein 15

Chicken and Broccoli Casserole

- » 18 oz. chicken breast, diced
- » 1 clove garlic, diced
- » 1/2 c. onion, diced
- » Salt and pepper
- » 2 c. broccoli, chopped
- » 1/2 lemon, juiced
- » 1/4 c. mayo with olive oil
- » 1/4 c. plain nonfat Greek yogurt
- » 1 c. wild rice, cooked
- » 3 oz. reduced-fat feta cheese

Cook rice and set aside one cup. Cook chicken breast, garlic, onion, salt, and pepper in nonstick pan over medium heat until juices run clear. Remove from heat. Combine all ingredients in a large bowl. Season with salt and pepper to taste. Spoon into nine-by-eleven-inch baking dish. Bake, uncovered, at 375 degrees for twenty-five minutes.

Serves four. Per Serving: calories 308, fat 10, carbs 16, protein 37

Turkey-Stuffed Acorn Squash

- 1/2 c. sun-dried tomato, hydrated
- 1/4 c. parmesan cheese, grated
- 3 Italian turkey sausages, casing removed
- 1 lb. ground turkey breast
- 3 T. garlic, minced
- 1/3 c. flaxseed, ground
- 1 egg
- 1/4 c. fresh basil, chopped
- 2 acorn squash

Heat oven to 350. In a large bowl, mix ground turkey breast with turkey sausage. Then chop the sun-dried tomatoes and add to turkey, along with garlic, basil, parmesan cheese, egg, and flaxseed. Halve the acorn squash, and remove seeds. Divide turkey mixture into four portions and form into balls, placing each in cavity of acorn squash. Place on a baking sheet lined with foil and bake for fifty to sixty minutes or until acorn squash pierces easily with a fork. Serve with side salad if desired. Enjoy

Serves four. Per Serving: calories 422, fat 23, carbs 25, protein 33.

Easy Beef Tenderloin with Sweet Potatoes

- 4 medium sweet potatoes
- 1 lb. fresh green beans
- 1 T. olive oil
- 4 6-oz. beef tenderloin steaks

Heat grill over medium-high heat and grill or broil steaks until desired doneness. Place foil on a sheet pan and bake sweet potatoes for thirty minutes at 350. Then toss green beans with a small amount of olive oil and add to sheet pan. Roast fifteen minutes or until tender. Serve each six-ounce tenderloin with one small sweet potato and green beans. (Can microwave potatoes and green beans if time is an issue.)

Serves four. Per Serving: calories 625, fat 38, carbs 36, protein 34.

Simple Turkey Tenderloin and Wild Rice

- 1 1/2 lb. turkey tenderloin
- 1 15-oz. can cooked wild rice, drained
- 4 c. broccoli florets

Season turkey tenderloins with low-sodium seasoning of choice. Heat grill over medium-high heat and grill turkey about seven minutes per side or until cooked through. Place rice in a microwave-safe dish and heat about ninety seconds. Place broccoli in a microwave-safe dish and add a small amount of water. Cook until desired doneness. Serve six ounces of turkey tenderloin with half a cup of rice and one cup of broccoli sprayed with I Can't Believe It's Not Butter spray or Bragg's Amino Acid.

Serves four. Per Serving: calories 371, fat 12, carbs 21, protein 43.

Quick and Easy Spicy Haddock

- 2 c. salsa
- 1 1/2 lb. frozen haddock filet, thawed
- 2 T. fresh cilantro, chopped

Preheat oven to 350 degrees. Rinse and dry fillets. Place fillets in a casserole dish coated with cooking spray. Pour salsa over fillets. Bake for twenty to thirty minutes until flakes easy with a fork. Sprinkle with cilantro. Serve over brown rice if desired.

Serves four. Per Serving: calories 187, fat 2, carbs 9, protein 34.

Blueberry Basil Poached Salmon

» 2 shallots, finely chopped

» 1 lb. salmon steak cut into 4-oz. portions

» 1 T. olive oil

» 2 T. fresh basil, chopped

» 1 T. honey

» 6 oz. fresh blueberries

» 2 T. balsamic vinegar

In a small skillet, heat olive oil over medium heat. Add shallots and sauté for three minutes. Stir in basil, honey, and vinegar. Simmer until mixture begins to thicken, stirring occasionally. Stir in blueberries and simmer for one minute. Pour into a bowl and cool. To poach salmon, use a large pot with enough water to cover steaks (adding a teaspoon of salt to water). Bring water to a boil and then lower heat to a simmer. Place salmon steaks in water and cook until desired doneness. Top poached salmon with blueberry basil sauce.

Serves four. Per Serving: calories 205, fat 7, carbs 11, protein 23.

Vegetarian Spinach Casserole

- » 1 c. reduced-fat cheddar cheese
- » 2 tsp. lemon juice
- » 1 c. low-fat cottage cheese
- » 2 tsp. onion powder
- » 2 T. parmesan cheese, grated
- » 7 whole eggs
- » 8 c. fresh baby spinach, cooked and drained
- » 2 tsp. dried basil
- » 1 c. cooked brown rice
- » 1/2 tsp. cayenne pepper
- » Pepper to taste

Preheat oven to 350 degrees. Mix three eggs, lemon juice, brown rice, basil, parmesan, and onion powder together to create layer one. Mix remaining ingredients together separate from the first layer. Spread the first-layer ingredients in the bottom of a greased casserole dish. Spread the second layer ingredients over the top. Bake for forty-five to sixty minutes.

Serves four. Per Serving: calories 316, fat 13, carbs 19, protein 30.

Cottage Cheese Meatloaf

- 1/2 c. rolled oats
- 1 T. prepared mustard
- 1/8 tsp. pepper
- 1/3 c. parmesan cheese, grated
- 2 T. onion, chopped
- 1/4 c. low-carb ketchup
- 1 lb. lean ground beef
- 1 egg lightly beaten
- 1 c. cottage cheese, small curd

In a bowl, combine cottage cheese, egg, ketchup, onions, mustard, rolled oats, and pepper. Add beef and mix well. Press into non-greased eight-inch-square baking pan. Bake at 350 degrees for twenty minutes. Sprinkle on parmesan and bake ten to fifteen minutes more until meat is no longer pink. Drain and let stand ten minutes before slicing.

Serves four. Per Serving: calories 415, fat 24, carbs 13, protein 35.

Quick and Simple Turkey Chili with Olive and Sun-Dried Tomato Tapenade

- 1/3 c. sun-dried tomatoes, packed in olive oil
- 1 1/2 tsp. pepper
- 1 T. olive oil
- 1 lb. lean ground turkey
- 1 head endive
- 2 tsp. garlic powder
- 1 can dark-red kidney beans
- 2 tsp. cumin
- 1 1/2 T. chili powder
- 8 oz. black olives, drained
- 1 tomato, diced

Quick & Simple Turkey Chili

Heat olive oil in a pot and add ground turkey. Brown turkey, and add garlic, chili powder, and cumin. Add beans and diced tomatoes, undrained. Simmer for one hour. Top with a tablespoon of low-fat sour cream, and sprinkle with reduced-fat cheese (optional).

Olive and Sun-Dried Tomato Tapenade

Place olives and sun-,dried tomatoes in a food processor and pulse until smooth. Gently pull endive leaves apart, wash and dry completely. Place small amount of tomato and olive mixture on endive leaves and enjoy.

Serves four. Per Serving: calories 351, fat 15, carbs 32, protein 25.

Buffalo Turkey Salad

- 24 oz. turkey breast meat, diced
- 1 clove garlic, diced
- 1/4 c. hot sauce
- 3 tsp. olive oil
- Salt and pepper
- 2 c. romaine lettuce, shredded
- 6 c. spinach
- 1 c. cherry tomatoes, halved
- 1/2 c. celery, chopped
- 1 c. carrots, chopped
- 1/4 red onion, thinly sliced
- 4 oz. reduced-fat feta cheese

Sauté turkey, garlic, hot sauce, olive oil, salt, and pepper in nonstick pan over medium-high heat for about three minutes. Remove from heat. Place lettuce in bowl and toss to combine. Top with chicken mixture, veggies, and cheese.

Serves four. Per Serving: calories 295, fat 10, carbs 15, protein 36.

Stuffed Red Peppers

» 1 1/4 c. dry quinoa
» 20 oz. extra-lean ground turkey
» 1 clove garlic, diced
» 1 1/2 T. olive oil
» 1/2 c. mushrooms, diced
» 1 c. canned tomatoes, drained
» 1/2 c. zucchini, diced
» Salt and pepper
» 2 tsp. tarragon
» 4 red bell peppers
» 3 T. parmesan cheese, grated

Cook quinoa and set aside. Sauté turkey, garlic, olive oil, mushrooms, tomatoes, zucchini, salt, and pepper in nonstick pan over medium-high heat until turkey is browned. Remove from heat and stir in quinoa and tarragon. Cut tops off peppers and remove ribs. Stuff peppers. Top with cheese. Bake at 375 degrees until cheese is brown and peppers are desired tenderness.

Serves four. Per Serving: calories 302, fat 9, carbs 19, protein 37.

Tuna and Broccoli Stir Fry

- » 1/2 lb. tuna steak, diced
- » 1 tsp. sesame oil
- » 1 scallion, chopped
- » 4 oz. pickled ginger
- » 2 tsp. hoisin sauce
- » 2 tsp. ginger, minced
- » 1 T. garlic, minced
- » 1/2 lb. fresh broccoli florets
- » 1 T. canola oil

Blanch broccoli in boiling water for five minutes and then drain. In a large skillet or wok, toss broccoli and tuna over medium-high heat with canola and sesame oil. Cook while stirring for three to four minutes. Add ginger root, pickled ginger, garlic, and hoisin sauce. Serve over brown rice if desired.

Serves two. Per Serving: calories 303, fat 15, carbs 11, protein 31.

Blackberry Chicken and White Bean Soup

» 1 T. olive oil

» 2 1/2 c. low-sodium chicken broth

» 1 lemon, sliced

» 1 dash garlic salt

» 1/4 tsp. fennel seed, crushed

» 1 tsp. dried basil

» 4 chicken breast, bone in

» 1 c. celery, finely chopped

» 1/2 c. carrot, peeled and diced

» 1 can cannellini beans, drained and rinsed

» 2 c. blackberries, washed and drained

» 1 tomato, diced

» 4 sprigs rosemary

» 1 c. onion, finely chopped

Blackberry Chicken

Preheat oven to 350 degrees. Carefully lift skin off of the chicken breast and stuff with one rosemary sprig, 1/4 cup of blackberries, and 1 slice of lemon. Sprinkle with garlic salt. Roast at 350 degrees for forty-five minutes or until juices run clear and golden brown.

White Bean Soup

In a large saucepan, heat olive oil over medium heat. Add onion, celery, carrots, and pepper. Sauté for five minutes. Add tomatoes, broth, basil, and fennel and bring to a boil. Cover, lower heat, and simmer for ten minutes. Add cannellini beans and simmer three minutes until beans are heated through.

Serves four. Per Serving: calories 440, fat 6, carbs 52, protein 47.

Slow Cooker Tomatillo Chicken

- 8 tomatillos, husked, rinsed, and sliced 1/4-inch thick
- 1/4 c. pickled jalapeno pepper, sliced
- 1 onion, thinly sliced
- 4 medium sweet potatoes, sliced 1/4-inch thick
- 2 T. jalapeno juice
- 1 T. garlic, minced
- 1/3 c. fresh cilantro, chopped
- 4 chicken breast, bone in

In a slow cooker, layer onion and then potato slices, chicken breasts, cilantro, garlic, and tomatillos. Sprinkle with salt, pepper, jalapeno slices, and jalapeno juice. Cover and slow cook on high for six hours. Remove chicken and place liquid from slow cooker in a pan. Boil down to reduce consistency of sauce. Pour sauce over each chicken breast.

Serves four. Per Serving: calories 312, fat 3, carbs 40, protein 31.

Simple Peanut Pork Tenderloin with Cabbage Rice

- » 1 lb. pork tenderloin, thinly sliced
- » 2 onions, thinly sliced
- » 2 T. olive oil
- » 1/2 c. natural peanut butter
- » 2 tsp. low-sodium soy sauce
- » 1/2 tsp. ground coriander
- » 1 T. garlic, minced
- » 1 tsp. dried red pepper
- » 1 bag cabbage, shredded
- » 1 can tomato sauce

Simple Peanut Pork Tenderloin

Preheat oven to 350 degrees. Arrange pork (can substitute chicken or turkey) in oven-proof baking dish. In a skillet, fry onion and garlic. Then add remaining ingredients, blending well. Pour sauce over pork and cover. Bake for thirty minutes and then remove cover and bake additional fifteen to twenty minutes or until done. Serve over cauliflower or cabbage rice.

Cabbage Rice

Boil two cups of water. Toss shredded cabbage with olive oil and desired spices. Place cabbage in a vegetable steamer. Steam for eight to ten minutes or until desired texture. Use tongs to sift through cabbage and ensure even doneness.

Use in place of rice in stir-fry or chicken dishes needing rice.

Serves four. Per Serving: calories 476, fat 24, carbs 28, protein 37

Poblano-Stuffed Peppers

- » 3 c. red enchilada sauce, no sugar added
- » 8 fresh poblano chili peppers
- » 4 chicken breasts, cooked and shredded
- » 1/4 c. black olive, sliced
- » 8 oz. reduced-fat Monterrey jack cheese

Preheat broiler. Broil peppers, turning until scorched on all sides. Remove from heat and place in paper bag and seal for ten minutes. Remove peppers and peel skin off. Make a slit down side and remove seeds. Turn oven down to 350 degrees. In a bowl, add shredded chicken, 1/2 cup cheese, and 1 cup enchilada sauce. Divide mixture, and stuff each pepper. Arrange peppers in a casserole dish and cover with remaining enchilada sauce. Bake thirty-five minutes until bubbly and then sprinkle with remaining cheese and bake five minutes. Garnish with olives and optional low-fat sour cream.

Serves four. Per Serving: calories 447, fat 21, carbs 14, protein 49

Grilled Salmon and Cucumber Salad

» 16 oz. salmon
» 1 lemon, juiced
» 1/4 c. balsamic vinegar
» 3 T. fresh chives, chopped
» 1 clove garlic, chopped
» Salt and pepper
» 2 c. cherry tomatoes, halved
» 2 c. cucumber, diced
» 1/2 c. red onion, sliced
» 3 T. Dijon mustard
» 1 c. plain nonfat Greek yogurt
» 1 green onion, diced

Place salmon on generous piece of aluminum foil. Turn edges up to form a boat. Squeeze half of the lemon juice onto the fish. Drizzle with balsamic vinegar. Scatter chives and garlic and season with salt and pepper. Grill until salmon is desired wellness. Stir together tomatoes, cucumbers, red onion, mustard, and Greek yogurt. Serve salmon over cucumber salad, and garnish with green onion.

Serves four. Per Serving: calories 295, fat 9., carbs 14, protein 36

Mediterranean Chicken and Soy Beans

» 1 tsp. white wine vinegar
» 2 tomatoes, chopped
» 1 tsp. red wine vinegar
» 8 pitted kalamata olives, halved
» 1/2 onion, chopped
» 2 T. olive oil
» 1 T. garlic clove, minced
» 1/4 c. fresh herb of choice, chopped
» 1 bunch fresh basil, chopped
» 4 chicken breast, bone in
» 1 15-oz. can soybeans

Preheat oven to 375 degrees. Place each chicken breast on a large square of aluminum foil. Combine one chopped tomato, half of onion, eight kalamata olives, 1 T. olive oil, 1 tsp. white wine vinegar, and the bunch of chopped basil in a bowl. Spoon over chicken. Fold foil up and seal to form a packet. Bake until chicken is cooked through, about twenty to thirty minutes.

For the beans, heat saucepan over medium heat and add 1 T. of olive oil. Add 1 T. of garlic and cook two minutes. Add soybeans, other chopped tomato, 1/4 cup of herbs, and 1 teaspoon of red wine vinegar. Cook five minutes until heated through.

Carefully open chicken packets and transfer to two plates. Serve with beans alongside chicken.

Serves four. Per Serving: calories 467, fat 23, carbs 23, protein 45.

Baked Avocados and Shrimp

- » 4 scallions, chopped
- » 8 raw shrimp, peeled and deveined
- » 1 tsp. mustard
- » 1/2 c. low-fat mayonnaise
- » 1/2 lemon, juiced
- » 1 hardboiled egg, chopped
- » 1 tsp. garlic
- » 2 avocados, halved, pitted, and peeled
- » 1/2 tsp. tarragon vinegar

Preheat oven to 350 degrees. Place in blender or food processor mayonnaise, garlic, mustard, egg, vinegar, and scallions. Pulse until well blended. Arrange cut avocados on a baking pan. Sprinkle with lemon juice. Place shrimp in depression left by pits. Cover liberally with blended sauce. Bake for twenty minutes or until shrimp is pink. Serve hot! Serve with a side salad if desired.

Serves four. Per Serving: calories 377, fat 24, carbs 15, protein 27.

Beef Tenderloin with Mushroom Wine Sauce and Broccoli Apple Salad

- » 3/4 tsp. pepper
- » 1/2 c. low-sodium beef broth
- » 1/2 c. onion, chopped
- » 8 oz. mushrooms, cleaned and sliced
- » 1/4 lb. Golden Delicious apples, diced
- » 1/2 tsp. garlic powder
- » 2 tsp. garlic
- » 1/4 c. dry red wine
- » 1 T. Dijon mustard
- » 2 tsp. cornstarch
- » 3 T. cider vinegar
- » 1 T. canola oil
- » 1 lb. broccoli floret
- » 4 5-oz. beef tenderloin steaks
- » 1 T. Splenda or stevia

Beef Tenderloin with Mushroom Wine Sauce

Sprinkle steaks with garlic powder and 1/4 tsp. pepper. Place a large nonstick skillet over medium-high heat until hot. Add steaks; cook three minutes on each side or until browned. Remove steaks from skillet and keep warm. Add mushrooms and fresh garlic to skillet. Cook, stirring constantly, for five minutes or until tender. Combine broth, wine, and cornstarch in a bowl, stirring until smooth. Add to skillet; cook, stirring constantly, for two minutes or until thick and bubbly. Return steaks and any steak juices to skillet and cook two additional minutes or until desired degree of doneness. Place each steak on a plate, and spoon mushrooms and sauce over steaks.

Broccoli Apple Salad

In a bowl, whisk together sweetener, remaining pepper, vinegar, oil, and mustard. Add chopped broccoli and toss. Then add apples and onion and toss again. Cover and chill at least one hour.

Serves four. Per Serving: calories 428, fat 30, carbs 14, protein 26.

Dijon Chicken with Healthy Ratatouille

» 4 chicken breasts
» 2 T. Dijon mustard
» 2 tsp. dried parsley
» 1/4 c. dry white wine
» 1 eggplant, cut into 1/2-inch cubes
» 2 T. garlic
» 1 T. garlic clove, minced
» 1 green bell pepper, chopped
» 2 c. mushrooms, cleaned and sliced
» 2 T. olive oil
» 1 onion, thinly sliced
» 1 c. parmesan cheese
» 2 tomato, chopped
» 1/2 tsp. Worcestershire sauce
» 2 zucchinis, sliced

Dijon Chicken

Heat one tablespoon oil in a large frying pan over medium-high heat. Add chicken and cook until golden, about three to four minutes per side. Remove chicken from pan and pour in wine (or water). Scrape up brown bits from pan to flavor the sauce. Stir in mustard, garlic, and Worcestershire sauce. Return chicken to pan and turn to coat. Cover and reduce heat to medium-low. Simmer, turning chicken occasionally, about eight to ten minutes.

Healthy Ratatouille

Preheat oven to 350 degrees. Coat a 1 1/2-quart casserole dish with cooking spray. Heat one tablespoon olive oil in a medium skillet over medium heat. Sauté garlic until lightly brown. Mix in parsley and eggplant. Sauté until soft, about ten minutes. Spread eggplant mixture evenly over bottom of prepared casserole dish. Sprinkle with a few tablespoons of parmesan cheese. Spread zucchini in an even layer over top. Sprinkle a little more cheese. Continue layering in this fashion with onion, mushrooms, bell pepper, and tomatoes, covering each layer with a sprinkling of cheese. Bake for forty-five minutes and enjoy!

Serves four. Per Serving: calories 367, fat 15, carbs 19, protein 40

Easy Beef and Cabbage Stew

- » 1 lb. lean ground beef
- » 2 tsp. Greek seasoning
- » 1 16-oz. package coleslaw mix
- » 1 15-oz. can pinto beans
- » 1 15-oz. can kidney beans
- » 1 14.5-oz. can of Italian-style diced tomatoes
- » 1 11.5-oz. can tomato juice
- » 1 10-oz. can diced tomatoes with green chili peppers
- » 1 1/2 c. water

In a large pot over medium heat, cook beef until brown; drain. Return meat to pot with pinto beans, kidney beans, diced tomatoes, tomato juice, water, coleslaw mix, and Greek seasoning. Simmer over low heat for one hour. Enjoy!

*Optional—ladle in bowl and serve with reduced-fat cheese sprinkled on top.

Serves eight. Per Serving: calories 314, fat 11, carbs 34, protein 22.

Italian Chicken Done Easy

» 1 T. olive oil
» 2 tsp. Italian seasoning
» 1 T. garlic
» 1 tsp. crushed red pepper
» 4 chicken breast
» 1 9-oz. package frozen green beans
» 1 28-oz. can stewed tomatoes, drained

In a large skillet, heat oil over medium-high heat. Add chicken, Italian seasoning, garlic, and crushed red pepper. Sauté for five minutes and then add tomatoes and cook for another five minutes. Add green beans and stir all together. Cover skillet, reduce heat to medium-low, and simmer approximately fifteen to twenty minutes.

Serves four. Per Serving: calories 195, fat 5, carbs 8, protein 29.

Pork Tenderloin and Acorn Squash

- 1/2 tsp. rosemary, dried
- 2 6-oz. pork tenderloins
- 1 T. olive oil
- 2 T. hoisin sauce
- 8 cloves of garlic, chopped
- 2 lb. acorn squash

Heat oven to 375 degrees. Scatter squash (quartered and sliced, skin on) in roasting pan. Mix rosemary, salt, and pepper. Rub into pork. Place in pan with squash and roast twenty-five minutes. Brush pork with hoisin sauce and continue roasting fifteen minutes until pork reaches an internal temperature of 140 degrees. Let meat stand five minutes before slicing.

Serves four. Per Serving: calories 379, fat 11, carbs 22, protein 48.

Tuna Steak with Veggies and Pine Nuts

» 2 6-oz. tuna steaks

» 3 T. tomato sauce

» 1 tsp. sesame oil

» 1 T. reduced-sodium soy sauce

» 1/4 c. pine nuts, toasted

» 1 T. olive oil

» 1/2 c. pea pod, chopped

» 1 c. Napa cabbage, shredded

» 1 tsp. lime juice

» 1/2 c. carrots, grated

Sauté vegetables with olive oil in a nonstick skillet over medium-high heat until crisp tender. Add tomato sauce and pine nuts, cook two minutes, and set aside. Set grill on medium-high heat. Mix sesame oil, lime juice, and soy sauce in a bowl. Rub mixture over tuna and grill for four minutes per side or until desired doneness is reached. Serve with veggies.

Serves two. Per Serving: calories 319, fat 17, carbs 11, protein 33

Grilled Chicken Pizza Packets

» 1 c. reduced-fat mozzarella cheese
» 1 red bell pepper, thinly sliced
» 1/2 c. parmesan cheese, grated
» 1/2 tsp. oregano, dried
» 1 onion, thinly sliced
» 1 T. olive oil
» 1 T. garlic, minced
» 1 tsp. dried basil
» 1 lb. chicken breast
» 16 soy pepperoni slices
» 1 zucchini, sliced

Cube chicken breasts. In a large mixing bowl, add chicken, olive oil, zucchini, soy pepperoni, red pepper, onion, garlic, and seasoning. Toss to combine. Coat four twelve-inch pieces of aluminum foil with cooking spray. Place 1/4 of mixture onto the center of each piece of foil. Fold foil around chicken mixture and seal tightly. Grill over medium-hot coals for twenty to twenty-five minutes or until chicken juices run clear. Open each packet and sprinkle with cheese and seal loosely. Grill an additional two minutes or until cheese melts.

Serves four. Per Serving: calories 393, fat 22, carbs 8, protein 39.

Red Snapper with Strawberry Avocado Salsa

» 2 c. strawberry

» 4 6-oz. red snapper fillets, with skin

» 1/4 c. red onion, chopped

» 1 T. olive oil

» 1 1/2 tsp. lime zest

» 1 T. lime juice

» 1 jalapeno pepper, minced

» 1/4 c. fresh cilantro, chopped

» 1 avocado, peeled, pitted, and diced

In a bowl, combine jalapeno, strawberries (finely chopped), red onions, cilantro, lime juice, and avocado and toss gently. Heat grill. Brush both sides of fish with olive oil. Sprinkle fish with lime zest. Grill fish, skin side down, without turning until cooked through; about eight to ten minutes. Transfer fish, skin side up, and remove skin carefully. Serve with strawberry salsa on top and a side salad (optional)! Enjoy!

Serves four. Per Serving: calories 312, fat 14, carbs 11, protein 37

Crab Salad with Orange Vinaigrette

» 3 c. orange juice, no sugar added
» 1 orange
» 1/2 c. olive oil
» 1 T. garlic clove, minced
» 1/4 c. fresh basil, finely sliced
» 2 lb. crabmeat, jumbo lump, shells removed
» 1/4 c. champagne vinegar
» 1/4 c. red onion, thinly sliced
» 1/2 c. walnut, toasted
» 2 T. fresh thyme
» 1 lb. baby spinach

Vinaigrette

Place a medium saucepan over medium-high heat, add orange juice, and reduce by half. Remove from heat and place in refrigerator to cool. Once orange reduction is cool, place in a mixing bowl with the champagne vinegar, olive oil, basil, thyme, and garlic. Season with salt substitute and pepper to taste. Set aside.

Salad

In a medium mixing bowl, combine spinach, toasted walnuts, orange (peeled, segmented, and chopped), and red onion. Place crab meat in the center of the salad. Drizzle vinaigrette over lightly and serve.

Serves six. Per Serving: calories 461, fat 25, carbs 21, protein 38.

Chicken Pumpkin Stew

- » 1 14.5-oz. can diced tomatoes
- » 1 1/2 lb. chicken breast
- » 1 T. cornstarch
- » 8 oz. fresh green beans
- » 1 T. garlic clove, minced
- » 14.5 oz. low-sodium chicken broth
- » 1/4 c. natural peanut butter
- » 1 T. olive oil
- » 1 onion, chopped
- » 1 red bell pepper, chopped
- » 1 T. smoked paprika
- » 3 c. sugar pumpkin or butternut squash

Heat oil in a large saucepan over medium-high heat. Add chicken (cut into cubes), sauté until brown, and move to a plate. Reduce heat to medium and add onions, red pepper, and garlic. Sauté four minutes until softened. Add 1 1/2 cups broth, tomatoes, and paprika. Bring to a boil and then add chicken, pumpkin (or squash), and beans. Reduce heat, cover, and simmer twelve minutes or until chicken and pumpkin are tender. Meanwhile stir remaining broth, cornstarch, and peanut butter in a bowl until smooth. Add to pot and stir until blended. Cook two minutes or until thickened and enjoy!

Serves four. Per Serving: calories 401, fat 13, carbs 28, protein 42.

Red Cabbage Turkey Stew

- » 1 poblano pepper, diced
- » 2 T. olive oil
- » 3 Italian turkey sausages, casing removed
- » 1 lb. ground turkey breast
- » 1 T. ground sage
- » 2 T. garlic, minced
- » 1/3 c. fresh basil, chopped
- » 1 4-oz. can green chilies, diced
- » 1 28-oz. can diced tomatoes, undrained
- » 1 15-oz. can tomato sauce
- » 1 15-oz. can lentils, drained
- » 1 15-oz. black soy beans, drained
- » 1 14.5-oz. can low-sodium chicken broth
- » 1 10-oz. bag shredded red cabbage

Heat a large pot over medium-high heat with olive oil. Sauté poblano and garlic until tender. Add ground turkey breast along with turkey sausage and cook through. Add the rest of the ingredients and simmer for thirty minutes. Optional: Serve with a dollop of low-fat sour cream or reduced-fat shredded cheese sprinkled on top.

Serves four. Per Serving: calories 464, fat 22, carbs 32, protein 36.

African Chicken Peanut Stew

- » 4 c. reduced-sodium chicken broth
- » 1 tsp. red pepper flakes
- » 1 red onion, chopped
- » 1/2 c. red bell pepper, chopped
- » 1 pumpkin or butternut squash, peeled, seeded, and diced
- » 1/2 c. natural peanut butter
- » 2 T. olive oil
- » 1 lemon, juiced
- » 2 tsp. ginger
- » 2 T. garlic, minced
- » 1 tsp. coriander
- » 1 tsp. cumin
- » 1 tsp. curry powder
- » 1/4 tsp. cinnamon
- » 1/2 c. cilantro, chopped
- » 2 lb. chicken breast, cubed
- » 1/2 c. celery, chopped
- » 1/4 c. carrots, peeled and diced
- » 1 acorn squash, peeled, seeded, and diced
- » 1 6-oz. can tomato paste
- » 1 tomato, chopped
- » 2 tsp. salt

This takes a bit of time but is well worth it for a nice evening meal. In a large sauté pan over medium-high heat, add 1 tablespoon olive oil and sauté chicken until opaque. In a large pot, heat 1 tablespoon olive oil over medium-high heat. Sauté onion for two minutes and then add pumpkin or squash. Sauté ten minutes. Then add chicken, chicken broth, celery, carrots, garlic, seasonings, and tomato paste. Bring to a boil and then lower heat to a slow simmer and cover. Cook for forty-five minutes. Stir in peanut butter and cook two minutes. Stir in tomato and red bell pepper and cook ten more minutes. Turn off heat and stir in lemon juice and cilantro. Indulge … it is well worth the wait!

Serves eight. Per Serving: calories 409, fat 24, carbs 20, protein.

Tier Two Snack Ideas

Peanut Butter and Celery Sticks

- » 2 celery stalks
- » 2 T. natural peanut butter

Spoon one tablespoon of peanut butter into each celery stick.

Serves one. Per Serving: calories 188, fat 16, carbs 5, protein 9.

Mexi Deviled Eggs

- » 1 tsp. cilantro, chopped
- » 1/8 tsp. cumin
- » 4 eggs, hard boiled
- » 1 tsp. low-fat sour cream
- » 1 T. salsa

Slice eggs lengthwise and remove the yolk. Place the yolks in a small bowl and mash, adding the remainder of the ingredients. Spoon mixture into egg whites and serve.

Serves two. Per Serving: calories 152, fat 10, carbs 1, protein 13.

String Cheese Snack

- 2 slices string cheese, low fat

Eat and enjoy!

Serves one. Per Serving: calories 98, fat 4, carbs 1, protein 14.

Berries and Nuts

- 1 oz. almonds
- 1/4 c. raspberries
- Splenda or stevia to taste

Mix together in a small bowl, sweeten to liking, and enjoy! You can also use you choice of seasonal berries as well as your choice of nuts

Serves one. Per Serving: calories 198, fat 14, carbs 11, protein 7.

Tuna Boats

- » 1 6-oz. can tuna in water, drained
- » 4 small cucumber, peeled
- » 1/2 c. reduced-fat cheddar cheese, shredded
- » 1 T. onion, chopped
- » 1/4 c. low-fat mayonnaise
- » 1 tsp. lemon juice
- » 2 T. dill pickle relish
- » 1/2 c. celery, diced

Cut cucumbers in half lengthwise and remove seeds. Slice a small amount off the bottom so cucumbers lie flat. Combine the rest of the ingredients in a bowl and spoon into cucumbers. Serve and enjoy!

Serves four. Per Serving: calories 192, fat 8, carbs 11, protein 19.

Nutty Yogurt

- 1 T. walnut, chopped
- 6 oz. sugar-free vanilla yogurt

Sprinkle walnuts on top of yogurt and enjoy!

Serves one. Per Serving: calories 98, fat 1, carbs 14, protein 8.

Snackin' Nutz

» 1 oz. almonds or any mixed nuts

Eat and enjoy!

Serves one. Per Serving: calories 167, fat 15, carbs 6, protein 6.

Quick Cottage Cheese Salad

- » 4 roma tomatoes, chopped
- » 2 c. low-fat cottage cheese
- » 2 green onion, chopped
- » 2 cucumbers, peeled, seeded, and chopped
- » 1/2 tsp. dried basil

In a medium bowl, mix all ingredients and chill until ready to serve.

Serves four. Per Serving: calories 132, fat 2, carbs 14, protein 16.

Peanut Butter Cottage Cheese

- » 2 T. natural peanut butter
- » 1 c. low-fat cottage cheese
- » 1/4 tsp. cinnamon
- » Splenda or stevia to taste

Blend all ingredients in a blender and serve. Add sweetener for taste as needed!

Serves two. Per Serving: calories 188, fat 9, carbs 6, protein 18.

Cajun Turkey Roll

- » 2 large lettuce leaves
- » 1 T. low-fat mayonnaise
- » 1/4 tsp. Cajun seasoning
- » 4 slices deli turkey breast

Mix mayonnaise and Cajun seasoning together. Place two slices of turkey meat on lettuce leaf and spread with half of mayonnaise mixture and roll up turkey in lettuce. Repeat. Add cucumber, tomato, onion, and alfalfa if so desired.

Serves two. Per Serving: calories 60, fat 3, carbs 5, protein 4.

Midday Vanilla Protein Smoothies

- » 1 c. vanilla soy milk, sugar free
- » 1/2 T. vanilla extract
- » 1/2 c. low-fat cottage cheese
- » 1/2 c. egg substitute (Egg Beaters)
- » 1/4 tsp. cinnamon, optional
- » Splenda or stevia to taste

Place all ingredients in a blender and blend until smooth. Add sweetener to liking. Add ice cubes (optional).

Serves two. Per Serving: calories 181, fat 10, carbs 6, protein 17

Hummus Boats

- 2 T. hummus dip (any flavor)
- 2 celery sticks

Spoon one tablespoon of hummus dip into each celery stick. Enjoy!

Serves one. Per Serving: calories 35, fat 0, carbs 4, protein 2.

Pudding Smoothie

- » 1 T. instant pudding mix, sugar free (any flavor)
- » 6 cubes of ice
- » 1/2 c. sugar-free vanilla yogurt
- » 1/2 c. vanilla soy milk, sugar free
- » Splenda or stevia to taste

Place all ingredients in a blender, mix for thirty seconds, and add ice to desired consistency.

Serves one. Per Serving: calories 145, fat 3, carbs 23, protein 8.

Pumpkin Smoothie

- » 1 T. Splenda or stevia
- » 1/2 c. pumpkin, canned
- » 1/2 tsp. pumpkin pie spice
- » 6 ice cubes
- » 1 c. vanilla soy milk, sugar free

Add all ingredients except ice to blender and blend for a few seconds. Add ice and blend on high until ice is crushed. Sweeten to taste.

Serves one. Per Serving: calories 130, fat 1, carbs 22, protein 10.

Snackin' Edamame Style

- 1 6-oz. spray bottle of Braggs Liquid Amino
- 1 16-oz. frozen bag edamame beans, soybeans

Preheat oven to 400. Place aluminum foil on a sheet pan and spray with cooking oil. Spread frozen edamame beans on pan, and spray liberally with Braggs Liquid Amino. Roast fifteen minutes, remove pan, and spray with Braggs again. Roast another fifteen minutes and enjoy a tasty protein snack!

Serves four. Per Serving: calories 110, fat 5, carbs 6, protein 11

Vanilla Peanut Butter Pudding

- » 1 T. Splenda or stevia
- » 1 T. nut (your choice), crushed
- » 1 T. natural peanut butter
- » 1/2 c. low-fat vanilla Greek yogurt

Put yogurt, peanut butter, and sweetener in a bowl. Mix well until smooth and creamy. Sprinkle crushed nuts over the top and enjoy!

Serves one. Per Serving: calories 165, fat 0, carbs 10, protein 12.

Hummus Deviled Eggs

- 1/2 c. hummus dip (any flavor)
- 6 eggs

Place six eggs in a pot and fill with enough water to cover. Bring water to a boil and cook for ten to twelve minutes. Drain pot and run cool water over eggs. Then chill. Remove shell and cut in half, removing and discarding yolks. Fill each cavity with 2 tsp. of hummus and enjoy.

Serves three. Per Serving: calories 146, fat 1, carbs 8, protein 10.

Chapter 7

The Lifestyle!

Welcome to Tier Three

Congratulations! You've done it. You've successfully reached your weight-loss goal. From this point forward, you will be maintaining your new healthy body weight while continuing to improve your health and quality of life. In tier three, we will again be adjusting your macronutrient divisions for maintenance while giving you more flexibility to indulge within guidelines. While working within tier three, your objective is to assume taking control of your newfound healthy lifestyle. During this tier, you are allowed moderate, responsible alcoholic consumption, but it is *not* recommended.

In the Lifestyle you will have recipes you can follow, a full "Food Breakdown List" to help start putting together your own meals, as well as the option to go out one or two times a week and indulge for one meal that day only in whatever you desire. Splurging in moderation will not hurt you and in fact can actually nudge your metabolism by shocking your body. So splurge but go right back to your new eating habits immediately after!

Warning: Splurging or cheat meals may result in a food hangover. A food hangover is very much like an alcohol hangover where you're nauseous and sluggish. Your body will no longer be used to all the processed foods, sugar, and saturated fat and may react to it in a very discomfiting way.

In the upcoming pages, you will see recipes labeled in sections: breakfast, lunch, dinner, and snacks. After this section, you will find a section called "Food Breakdown List." This section will be packed full of all the foods I use in my recipes broken down into sections so you can start piecing together your own meals and recipes. Follow my guidelines and notations to assist you.

Try to eat approximately every three hours, and do not skip meals. Along with your meals, as well as throughout the day, you will need to take in a minimum of two quarts of water. This will continually help flush toxins from your body while keeping you adequately hydrated.

Other allowable beverages are as followed:

Note: A serving equals eight ounces.

» *water, water, water!*
» decaffeinated coffees and teas
» Crystal Light
» sugar-free Kool-Aid
» vegetable juices (no sugar)
» regular coffee and caffeinated diet soda (limit two servings a day)
» skim milk, 1 percent milk, soy milk, almond milk (limit two servings a day)

NOTE: I encourage you to maneuver back and forth throughout all three tiers from time to time. This will ensure your continued success without letting old bad habits slowly start creeping back into your life unexpectedly.

Tier Three Breakfast Recipes

Cheesy Ham and Turkey Hash Browns

» 1 1/4 c. organic hash browns
» 1 clove garlic, diced
» 1/2 c. onion, chopped
» 1/2 c. mushrooms, diced
» 2 c. extra lean ham, diced
» 8 oz. extra-lean turkey breast, diced
» Salt and pepper
» 1/2 c. reduced-fat cheddar cheese, shredded

Cook hash browns, garlic, onions, mushrooms, ham, turkey, salt, and pepper, in nonstick pan over medium-high heat for about ten minutes. Top with cheese.

Serves four. Per Serving: calories 311, fat 11, carbs 22, protein 28.

Protein Pancake and Turkey Bacon

- 1/3 c. egg whites
- 1/3 c. 1 percent cottage cheese
- 1/3 c. oatmeal
- 1 tsp. cinnamon
- 2 oz. organic low-fat turkey bacon

Combine the first four ingredients in a blender. Blend until smooth. Heat a small, nonstick pan over medium heat. Pour mixture into pan. Cover with lid. When top of pancake is set completely, flip. Cook the second side for one minute. Remove from pan. Cook turkey bacon until warm. Serve together.

Serves one. Per Serving: calories 312, fat 10, carbs 22, protein 31.

Egg Sandwich

- 1 100 percent whole wheat sandwich thin
- 2 organic eggs
- 3/4 c. egg whites
- Fresh chives, chopped
- Garlic powder
- Onion powder
- Salt and pepper

Whisk together eggs and egg whites. Add chives and seasonings. Cover eggs and cook eggs in nonstick pan over medium-high heat until set. Fold over and serve on sandwich thin.

Serves one. Per Serving: calories 300, fat 11, carbs 22, protein 29.

Breakfast Burrito

- » 3 c. egg whites
- » 1 c. black beans, drained and rinsed
- » 1/4 c. diced green chilies
- » 1 T. jalapeño, diced
- » 1 T. ground cumin
- » Salt and pepper
- » 4 low-carb tortillas
- » 1/2 c. salsa
- » Hot sauce
- » 32 almonds

Combine eggs, beans, jalapeño, and seasonings. Cook eggs in nonstick pan over medium-high heat, stirring constantly. Divide eggs among tortillas. Serve with salsa, hot sauce (if desired), and almonds.

Serves four. Per Serving: calories 261, fat 7, carbs 25, protein 29.

Blueberry and Peanut Butter Smoothie

- » 6 oz. plain, nonfat Greek yogurt
- » 1/2 c. fresh blueberries
- » 1 1/2 T. natural peanut butter
- » Water

Combine all ingredients in a blender using as much water as necessary.

Serves one. Per Serving: calories 298, fat 12, carbs 21, protein 24.

Protein Shake and Peanut Butter and Raspberry Pita

» 1/2 100 percent whole wheat pita pocket

» 1 T. natural peanut butter

» 1/4 c. raspberries, mashed

» 1 scoop 100 percent whey protein powder

» Water

Toast pita pocket and spread with peanut butter and raspberries. Shake protein powder and water until well blended.

Serves one. Per Serving: calories 335, fat 10, carbs 26, protein 31.

Oatmeal and Egg Twist

» 4 egg whites
» 1 c. water
» 1/2 c. old-fashioned rolled oats
» 1 tsp. cinnamon

Combine oats, egg whites, water, and cinnamon in a microwave-safe bowl. Microwave for about four minutes in one-minute increments, stirring in between. Let sit for about one minute and add Splenda or stevia and more cinnamon to taste. Top with two tablespoons of crushed walnuts if desired.

Serves one. Per Serving: calories 228, fat 3, carbs 30, protein 21.

Oat and Cashew Waffles

- » 2 T. old-fashioned rolled oats
- » 1/2 c. cashews
- » 1 T. canola oil
- » 1 c. water

Using a food processor or a blender, grind together the oats and cashews. Be careful not to over-grind or you will get a butter-like consistency. Add the oil and water and blend thoroughly. Pour the batter into a waffle iron and leave a few minutes until cooked. This recipe can also be cooked like a regular pancake. Serve with sugar-free syrup.

Serves four. Per Serving: calories 279, fat 14, carbs 32, protein 9.

Egg Salad and Crackers

- » 6 egg whites
- » 2 tsp. Dijon mustard
- » 1 T. pickled relish
- » 2 T. mayo with olive oil
- » 1 T. fresh dill, chopped
- » 1 T. fresh chives, chopped
- » 1 T. red onion, chopped
- » 1 T. lemon juice
- » Onion powder
- » Salt and pepper
- » 4 Triscuit crackers

Place eggs in a large pot of water. Bring to a boil. Place lid on pot and turn off burner. Leave eggs for nine minutes. Remove eggs and cool them. Shell them and remove the yolks. Mash eggs and combine them with remaining ingredients. Eat with crackers.

Serves one. Per Serving: calories 317, fat 11, carbs 22, protein 30.

Canadian Bacon and Broccoli Omelet

- 2 c. broccoli, chopped
- 2 slices organic low-fat Canadian bacon
- 1 c. cherry tomatoes, diced
- 1/2 c. onion, diced
- 1 clove garlic, diced
- Salt and pepper
- 4 eggs
- 1 c. egg whites
- 1 c. reduced-fat cheddar cheese
- 4 slices 100 percent whole wheat bread (15 g carbs)

Cook broccoli, Canadian bacon, tomatoes, onion, garlic, salt, and pepper in nonstick pan over medium-high heat for about five to seven minutes. Remove from pan. Whisk eggs together and season with salt and pepper. Pour 1/4 of the egg mixture into nonstick pan, cover, and cook over medium-high heat until set. Disperse 1/4 of the vegetable mixture onto 1/2 of the eggs. Top with 1/4 of the cheese. Fold egg over cheese, and repeat for remaining omelets.

Serves four. Per Serving: calories 308, fat 9, carbs 23, protein 29.

Cashew Waffles and Canadian Bacon

» 1/2 c. cashews

» 2 c. rolled oats

» 8 slices Canadian bacon

» 1 c. water

In a food processor or blender, grind oats and cashews. Don't over-grind or it will turn into a butter-like consistency. Add water and blend thoroughly. Spray waffle iron with cooking spray, and pour batter in. Cook a few minutes and serve with Canadian bacon and sugar-free maple syrup.

Serves four. Per Serving: calories 338, fat 14, carbs 33, protein 21.

Tier Three Lunch Recipes

Open-Faced Tuna Melt

- 12 oz. canned tuna in water, drained
- 1/2 c. mayo with olive oil
- 1/2 c. plain, nonfat Greek yogurt
- 1/2 c. Dijon mustard
- 1 c. celery, diced
- 1 c. reduced-fat cheddar cheese
- Salt and pepper
- 4 slices 100 percent whole wheat bread (15 g carbs)

Combine all ingredients except bread. Divide tuna mixture, and spread onto bread. Place bread onto indoor griddle and tent with foil. Remove when the bread is browned and the cheese is melted.

Serves one. Per Serving: calories 339, fat 11.5, carbs 22.9, protein 30.9.

Pepper-Encrusted Flank Steak and Sweet Potato

- 20 oz. flank steak
- 6-pepper blend
- 4 medium sweet potatoes
- Salt and pepper

Sprinkle six-pepper blend onto top side of each steak. Place steaks on *hot* grill, pepper side down to sear. Turn steaks and continue grilling until desired wellness. Bake sweet potatoes in a 375-degree oven until fork tender, about thirty minutes. Cut open and season with salt and pepper.

Serves four. Per Serving: calories 321, fat 10, carbs 23, protein 31.

Mexican Shrimp Salad

» 16 oz. raw shrimp
» 1 T. red pepper flakes
» 1 T. ground cumin
» 1 T. chili powder
» 1 T. garlic powder
» 1 T. onion powder
» 1/2 T. oregano
» 1/2 T. black pepper
» 1/2 T. sea salt
» 1 1/2 T. olive oil
» 1 can diced green chilies
» 1 clove garlic
» 12 c. spinach
» 1 c. cherry tomatoes, halved
» 1 c. corn
» 1 c. black beans, drained and rinsed
» 1 c. plain, nonfat Greek yogurt

Combine dry seasonings in small blender or with mortar and pestle. Sauté shrimp, dry seasonings, olive oil, garlic, and green chilies in nonstick pan over medium-high heat for about seven minutes or until shrimp are no longer translucent. Place spinach in large bowl. Top with shrimp and remaining ingredients.

Serves four. Per Serving: calories 282, fat 7, carbs 24, protein 31.5.

Chicken Sausage and Pasta Salad

- » 1 1/2 c. cooked organic pasta
- » 20 oz. organic, low-fat chicken sausage, sliced
- » 1/2 c. onion, chopped
- » 1 c. mushrooms, chopped
- » 1/2 T. fresh rosemary, chopped
- » 1/2 c. cherry tomatoes, diced
- » 2 T. capers
- » 2 cloves garlic, pressed
- » Salt and pepper
- » 1/2 lemon, juiced
- » Red pepper flakes
- » Parsley

Cook pasta and set aside 1 1/2 cups. Cook chicken sausage, onion, mushroom, rosemary, tomatoes, capers, garlic, salt, and pepper in nonstick pan over medium-high heat for about seven minutes. Combine pasta, chicken-sausage mixture, lemon juice, red pepper flakes, and parsley.

Serves four. Per Serving: calories 304, fat 10, carbs 21.4, protein 31.

Chicken and White Bean Salad

» 3 oz. chicken breast, grilled
» 3 c. spring mix lettuce
» 1/4 c. zucchini, sliced
» 1/4 c. white beans (great northern), drained and rinsed
» 1 oz. reduced-fat feta cheese
» 1 T. fresh basil, chopped
» 1/2 T. olive oil
» 2 T. ginger balsamic vinegar
» 1 fl. oz. orange juice
» Fresh black pepper

Grill chicken breast. Place greens in bowl. Top lettuce with chicken, zucchini, beans, feta cheese, and basil. Whisk together remaining ingredients to make dressing and pour over salad.

Serves one. Per Serving: calories 326, fat 12, carbs 23, protein 30.

Kicked-Up Shrimp Guacamole with Pita

» 20 oz. raw shrimp
» 1 T. olive oil
» 3 limes, juiced (about 1/2 c)
» 2 cloves garlic
» Salt and pepper
» 1/2 c. corn
» 1/2 c. red onion, diced
» 1/2 c. cherry tomatoes, diced
» 1 jalapeño, diced
» 1 avocado, diced
» Fresh cilantro, chopped
» 1 1/2 pita pockets, cut in pieces, baked if desired

Sauté shrimp, olive oil, lime juice, garlic, salt, and pepper in nonstick pan over medium-high heat for about seven minutes or until shrimp are no longer translucent. Remove from heat and cut shrimp into smaller pieces. Place in bowl. Stir in remaining ingredients and serve with pita pockets.

Serves four. Per Serving: calories 327, fat 12, carbs 25, protein 31.

Italian Chicken Sandwich

- 4 oz. chicken breast
- 1 tsp. olive oil
- Pinch oregano
- Pinch basil
- Pinch ground fennel
- Salt and pepper
- 2 T. tomato sauce
- 1 light string cheese, shredded
- 1 100 percent whole wheat sandwich thin

Sauté chicken breast and olive oil in nonstick pan over medium heat until juices run clear. Season with dry seasonings. Top with tomato sauce and cheese. Serve on sandwich thin.

Serves one. Per Serving: calories 301, fat 10, carbs 25, protein 31.

Thai Chicken Wrap

» 16 oz. chicken breast, shredded
» 2 T. soy sauce
» 2 limes, juiced
» 2 T. natural peanut butter
» 1 clove garlic
» Salt and pepper
» 4 slices light Flat Out bread
» 1/2 c. carrots, shredded
» 1/2 c. red cabbage, shredded
» 10 almonds, chopped

Heat shredded chicken in nonstick pan over medium heat, along with soy sauce, lime juice, peanut butter, garlic salt, and pepper, for five minutes. Remove from heat. Divide chicken among flat breads. Top with carrots, cabbage, and almonds.

Serves four. Per Serving: calories 312, fat 10, carbs 22, protein 32.

Jicama Chicken Salad

- 4 cooked chicken breasts
- 1/2 jicama, peeled and sliced into matchstick slices
- 3 navel oranges, peeled and sliced thin
- 1 bag romaine lettuce greens
- 1/4 c. toasted pecans, chopped
- 1/4 c. olive oil
- 2 T. red wine vinegar
- 1 tsp. honey
- 1 tsp. garlic, minced

In a bowl, mix chopped pecans, olive oil, red wine vinegar, honey, and garlic. In a second bowl, toss jicama, oranges, and greens. Portion greens onto plates and top each with a sliced chicken breast. Top with dressing mixture from first bowl.

Serves four. Per Serving: calories 381, fat 20, carbs 22, protein 30.

Quick Crab Gumbo

» 32 oz. reduced-sodium chicken broth

» 1 onion, chopped

» 1 T. olive oil

» 1 T. garlic

» 1 lb. frozen cut okra, defrosted and drained

» 2 tsp. creole seasoning

» 1 lb. crab meat or shrimp

» 2 c. cooked brown rice

» 2/3 c. tomato paste

Sauté onion and garlic until softened in a pot over medium-high heat. Slice okra and add to pot. Cook until tender. Add the rest of the ingredients except rice. Cook for thirty minutes, stirring occasionally. Serve with rice.

Serves four. Per Serving: calories 389, fat 6, carbs 45, protein 41.

Tier Three Dinner Recipes

Fish Tacos

- 12 oz. tilapia
- 1 1/2 T. olive oil
- Salt and pepper
- 8 100 percent whole wheat low-carb tortillas
- 1/2 red bell pepper, thinly sliced
- 1/4 red onion, thinly sliced
- 1/2 c. plain nonfat Greek yogurt
- 1/2 c. salsa
- 2 T. fresh cilantro, chopped
- 1/2 jalapeño, diced

Sauté tilapia and olive oil in nonstick pan over medium heat, gently flipping when lightly browned. Divide fish among tortillas. Top with pepper and onion. Combine yogurt, salsa, cilantro, and jalapeño, and top each taco with mixture.

Serves four. Per Serving: calories 263, fat 11, carbs 24, protein 30.

Curry Shrimp and Rice

» 2 1/2 c. wild rice, cooked
» 18 oz. raw shrimp
» 2 1/2 T. olive oil
» 2 cloves garlic, pressed
» 2 shallots, sliced
» Salt and pepper
» 1/2 c. plain, nonfat Greek yogurt
» 1–2 T. curry powder
» 1 T. fresh cilantro, chopped

Cook rice and set 2 1/2 cups aside. Sauté shrimp, olive oil, garlic, shallot, salt, and pepper in nonstick pan over medium-high heat for about seven minutes or until shrimp are no longer translucent. Remove from heat and immediately add rice and remaining ingredients.

Serves four. Per Serving: calories 310, fat 10, carbs 23, protein 30.

Cashew and Chicken Pasta Salad

- » 1 c. organic pasta, cooked
- » 12 oz. canned low-fat chicken, drained well
- » 1 c. celery, chopped
- » 1/2 c. green bell pepper, chopped
- » 1/2 c. yellow bell pepper, chopped
- » 1/2 c. red onion, chopped
- » 1/4 c. Dijon mustard
- » 1 c. plain, nonfat Greek yogurt
- » 1/2 T. fresh thyme
- » 1 T. dry ranch seasoning
- » 1/4 c. sunflower seeds
- » 1/4 c. cashew halves, chopped
- » Salt and pepper

Cook pasta and set aside one cup. Combine all ingredients and refrigerate for an hour or more.

Serves four. Per Serving: calories 323, fat 10, carbs 22, protein 30.

Mushroom and Rosemary Steak with Rice

- » 2 1/4 c. wild rice blend
- » 16 oz. round steak
- » Salt and pepper
- » 2 c. various mushrooms, chopped
- » 1/2 c. onion, chopped
- » 1 T. rosemary, chopped
- » 1 clove garlic, chopped
- » Pinch or two red pepper flakes
- » 1 1/2 T. olive oil

Cook rice and set aside 2 1/4 cups. Season steaks with salt and pepper on both sides, and grill to desired wellness. Let steak sit for three to five minutes. Sauté mushrooms, onions, rosemary, garlic, red pepper flakes, salt, pepper, and olive oil in nonstick pan over medium heat for five minutes. Cut steak into strips. Serve steak over rice, and top with mushrooms and onions.

Serves four. Per Serving: calories 304, fat 10, carbs 22, protein 30.

Chicken Fajitas

- » 10 oz. chicken breast
- » 1 clove garlic, chopped
- » 1 bell pepper, sliced
- » 1/2 onion, sliced
- » 1 T. olive oil
- » Salt and pepper
- » 1 packet fajita seasoning
- » 4 100 percent whole wheat tortillas (18 g carbs)
- » 1/2 c. reduced-fat cheddar cheese
- » 1/2 c. plain, nonfat Greek yogurt

Sauté chicken breast, garlic, pepper, onion, olive oil, salt, and pepper in nonstick pan over medium heat until juices run clear. Add fajita seasoning and cook an additional five minutes. Add water if necessary. Divide chicken and veggies among tortillas. Top with cheese and yogurt.

Serves four. Per Serving: calories 254, fat 9, carbs 24, protein 29.

Pasta and Meatballs

- 1 c. pasta, cooked
- 3 oz. ground round
- 2 cloves of garlic, minced
- 10 oz. extra-lean ground turkey
- 1/3 c. panko bread crumbs
- 1/4 c. onion, diced
- 1 oz. Romano cheese
- 1 egg
- Salt and pepper
- 2 c. marinara sauce
- 1 T. fresh basil, chopped
- 1 T. fresh parsley, chopped

In large bowl, combine all ingredients but pasta and sauce. Form into meatballs of relatively equal size. Brown meatballs in nonstick pan over medium heat, turning to brown all sides. Add sauce and herbs and turn down heat. Simmer for ten minutes. Season with salt and pepper to taste.

Serves 4. Per Serving: calories 316, fat 10, carbs 25, protein 28.

Moroccan Chicken

» 1 zucchini, sliced
» 1/4 tsp. turmeric
» 1 c. tomato, chopped
» 2 stalk celery, thinly sliced
» 1 1/2 c. reduced-sodium chicken broth
» 1/2 tsp. paprika
» 1/2 tsp. oregano
» 1 onion, chopped
» 1 T. lemon juice
» 1 T. ginger root, minced
» 1 T. garlic clove, minced
» 1 tsp. cumin
» 1 lb. chicken breast
» 1/4 tsp. cayenne pepper
» 2 carrots, peeled and diced
» 1 c. canned chickpeas, drained

Brown cubed chicken in a large saucepan over medium heat until almost cooked through. Remove chicken and set aside. Sauté onion, garlic, carrots, and celery in the same pan. When tender, add ginger, paprika, cumin, oregano, cayenne, and turmeric. Sauté for one minute. Mix in broth and tomatoes. Return chicken to pan, reduce heat to low, and simmer ten minutes. Add chickpeas and zucchini and bring back to simmer. Cover pan and cook fifteen minutes or until zucchini is tender. Stir in lemon juice and serve.

Serves four. Per Serving: calories 277, fat 3, carbs 34, protein 31.

Pork Chops and Mashed Potatoes

- » 12 oz. pork loin chops
- » 2 T. organic bread crumbs
- » 2 tsp. olive oil
- » 2 c. green beans
- » 9 oz. red potatoes
- » 1/4 c. chicken broth
- » 1/4 c. plain, nonfat Greek yogurt
- » 1 leek, chopped
- » Garlic powder
- » Salt and pepper
- » 1 T. fresh parsley, chopped
- » 1 T. fresh chives, chopped

Place pork chops in baking dish. Combine olive oil and bread crumbs in dish and divide among chops. Bake at 375 degrees until no longer pink in the middle, about twenty minutes. Steam green beans and season with salt and pepper. Cut potatoes into equal pieces, and boil until fork tender. Drain and place in bowl. Stir remaining ingredients into potatoes.

Serves four. Per Serving: calories 297, fat 10, carbs 22, protein 28.

Teriyaki Shrimp and Mango Hummus Salsa

» 2 c. wild rice, cooked

» Wooden skewers

» 20 oz. raw shrimp

» 1/4 c. teriyaki sauce

» 1 mango, diced

» 1/2 c. cherry tomatoes, diced

» 1/2 c. red onion, chopped

» 1 clove garlic, chopped

» 1 lime, juiced

» 2 T. diced green chilies

» 2 T. original hummus

» Salt and pepper

» Fresh cilantro

Cook rice and set aside two cups. Soak skewers in water for twenty minutes. Slide shrimp on skewers. Grill shrimp on indoor grill, brushing with teriyaki frequently, until shrimp are no longer translucent. Remove from grill and set aside. Combine remaining ingredients to make salsa. Serve shrimp over rice with salsa on top. Garnish with cilantro.

Serves four. Per Serving: calories 312, fat 9, carbs 25, protein 32.

Saucy Chicken

- » 6 oz. tomato paste
- » 14 oz. spaghetti sauce, no sugar added
- » 16 oz. salsa, no sugar added
- » 1/3 c. parmesan cheese
- » 1 T. dried oregano
- » 1 T. dried thyme
- » 1 T. dried parsley
- » 6 chicken breasts
- » 1 1/2 c. brown rice
- » 1 10-oz. can whole tomatoes
- » 3 c. water

In a large pot over medium-low heat, mix together spaghetti sauce, salsa, tomatoes, tomato paste, parmesan, and seasonings. Place the chicken in a separate pot with enough water to cover. Bring to a boil, reduce heat to low, and simmer for twenty-five minutes, until chicken juices run clear. Transfer chicken to pot with sauce mixture. Cover and cook on low for one hour. In a separate pot, bring uncooked rice and water to a boil. Reduce heat to low, cover, and simmer for twenty minutes. Serve chicken and sauce over the cooked rice. Optional: Serve over spaghetti squash strands or cauliflower rice instead of brown rice.

Serves six. Per Serving: calories 427, fat 8, carbs 51, protein 37.

Food Breakdown List

Are you creative in the kitchen? An aspiring chef? Or do you have days when your schedule is so hectic that you just find it impossible to prepare a meal laid out in my book? These are the times when pre-cooked meats, poultry and fish, pre-made hardboiled eggs, bagged lettuce, and pre-cut or frozen veggies are going to come to the rescue and save you time while keeping you on track. Follow these simple guidelines when taking meal planning into your own hands:

» Base all protein (meats, poultry, and fish) serving sizes on your closed hand—about one inch thick. Make sure you have at least one serving with every meal!

» If eating hardboiled eggs as your protein source, three eggs are equivalent to one serving size.

» Make sure you get at least one cup of cooked or raw vegetables per meal.

» Follow the tier specifications when choosing foods from our starches, dairy, and fruit groups.

» Remember your snacks between meals.

» Drink plenty of water throughout the day and with meals in addition to other beverages.

Now for all you do-it-yourselfers, here is a food breakdown list of all the foods and ingredients used in my meal plans. It's even broken down by tier, so you can easily see which ingredients you are able to use at your specific stage ... Now get creative

Proteins

- » A serving size is equal to your fist—one-inch thick.
- » ground beef (96 percent lean)
- » ground round
- » ground sirloin
- » eye of round
- » flank steak
- » London broil
- » sirloin
- » T-bone
- » tenderloin
- » top loin
- » top round

Seafood

All types of fish and shellfish, including water-packed tuna and other canned fish.

Poultry

- » chicken breast (skinless)
- » ground chicken breast
- » ground chicken (lean)
- » turkey breast tenderloin
- » ground turkey breast
- » ground turkey (lean)
- » rotisserie chicken (no skin)

Pork

» pork loin
» pork tenderloin
» center-cut chops
» loin chops
» cutlets
» top round

Wild Game

» bison
» elk
» venison

Eggs

» whole eggs (no limit, unless directed by your doctor)
» egg whites and egg substitutes (no limit)

Deli Meats

» Note: Look for natural, nitrate-free meats.
» turkey slices
» chicken slices
» roast beef slices
» ham slices

Soy Meat Alternatives

» burger
» sausage
» hot dogs
» tofu (all varieties)
» yuba (bean curd or sheets)

Milk and Dairy

- fat-free or low fat, 1 percent or 2 percent only
- all tiers cottage cheese (fat-free or 1 percent to 2 percent, serving size 1/2 cup)
- cream cheese substitute (dairy free)
- low-fat milk (fat free or 1 percent)
- low-fat soy milk (no sugar added, make sure it does not contain high fructose corn syrup or maltodextrin)
- low-fat or nonfat yogurt (no sugar added, artificially sweetened)

Vegetables

- artichokes
- asparagus
- bok choy
- broccoli
- brussels sprouts
- cabbage
- capers
- cauliflower
- celery
- collard greens
- cucumbers
- eggplant
- green Beans
- leeks
- lettuce (all varieties)
- mushrooms (all varieties)
- okra

- » onions (all varieties)
- » peppers (all varieties)
- » pickles (dill or artificially sweetened)
- » radishes (all varieties)
- » snap peas
- » spinach
- » spaghetti squash
- » summer squash
- » tomatoes (all varieties)
- » water chestnuts
- » wax beans
- » zucchini

Carbohydrates

- » whole grain, stone-ground wheat or rye—one slice
- » whole oat, bran, multigrain, or pumpernickel—one slice
- » coarse European-style, sprouted whole wheat—one slice
- » 100 percent whole grain (low carb preferred)—one slice
- » stone-ground or whole wheat—1/2
- » high-fiber types like All Bran or Fiber One—1 cup
- » coarse oatmeal (slow cooked)—1/2 c. cooked
- » coarse whole grain (Kashi)—1/2 c. cooked
- » pasta (whole wheat or soy only)—1/2 c. cooked
- » brown, wild, or Basmati rice—1/2 c. cooked
- » beans (all varieties)—1/2 c. cooked
- » split peas and soy beans—1/2 c. cooked
- » sweet potato or yam—1 small

Fruits

- » apple (all varieties)—1
- » berries (all varieties)—1/2 cup
- » cantaloupe—3/4 cup
- » cherries—3/4 cup
- » grapefruit —1/2
- » grapes (all varieties)—3/4 cup
- » honeydew—3/4 cup
- » orange—1
- » peach—1
- » pear—1
- » plum—1 large or 2 small
- » tangerine—1
- » **Nuts and Seeds**
- » almonds
- » brazil nuts
- » cashews
- » flax seed (3 tablespoons)
- » hazelnuts
- » macadamia
- » peanuts
- » pecans
- » pine nuts
- » pistachios
- » sesame seeds
- » soy nuts
- » walnuts
- » natural peanut butter and other nut butter (2 tablespoons a day)

Oils

- » olive oil
- » canola oil
- » nonfat cooking spray (olive or canola)
- » smart Balance butter and products
- » I Can't Believe It's Not Butter (spray)
- » low-fat mayonnaise
- » olive oil, lime, or vinegar-based salad dressing (preferred)
- » spray dressing with 3 grams or less sugar per serving

Herbs and Spices

- » almond, vanilla, and other extracts
- » espresso powder
- » horseradish (sauce)
- » mustard
- » lemon and lime juice
- » pepper (all types)
- » salsa (no sugar added)
- » allspice
- » basil
- » bay leaf
- » cayenne
- » caraway seed
- » chilies (dried)
- » chili Powder
- » chives
- » cider Vinegar
- » cilantro

- cinnamon
- coriander
- cumin
- curry Powder
- dill
- garlic (not garlic salt)
- ginger
- mace
- marjoram
- nutmeg
- onion powder (not onion salt)
- paprika
- parsley
- pimiento
- poultry seasoning
- rosemary
- sage
- savory
- thyme
- turmeric

Artificial Sweeteners

- Stevia (preferred)
- Splenda (okay but not preferred)

Beverages

- *Note*: A serving equals eight ounces
- *water, water, water!*
- decaffeinated coffees and teas

» Crystal Light
» sugar-free Kool-Aid
» vegetable juices (no sugar)
» regular coffee and caffeinated diet soda (limit 2 servings a day)
» skim milk, 1 percent milk, soy milk, almond milk (tiers two and three only—limit two servings a day)